TEXT BOOK OF ENT AND MOUTH DISORDERS INCLUDING GASTROINTESTINAL ASSESSMENT

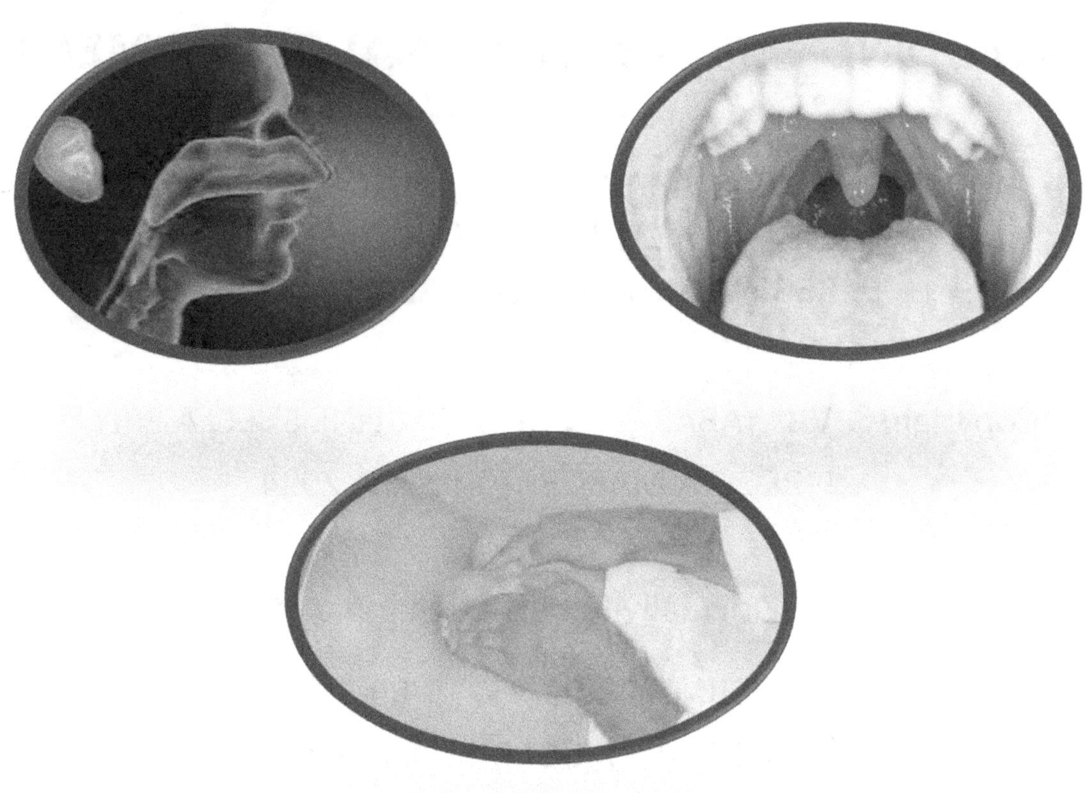

VIJAYABARATHI. M, M.SC(N)

S. PAULINE SHEELA PRIYA, M.SC(N)

J. REGINA MARGRET VIMALA, M.SC(N)

RIGI PUBLICATION

TEXT BOOK OF ENT AND MOUTH DISORDERS INCLUDING GASTROINTESTINAL ASSESSMENT

VIJAYABARATHI. M, M.SC(N)
S. PAULINE SHEELA PRIYA, M.SC(N)
J. REGINA MARGRET VIMALA, M.SC(N)

Originally Published in India

ISBN: 978-93-95773-80-5

Published by **RIGI PUBLICATION**

Printer: **Rigi printers**

777, Street no.9, Krishna Nagar

Khanna-141401 (Punjab), India

Website: www.rigipublication.com

Email: info@rigipublication.com

Phone: +91-9357710014, +91-9465468291

PREFACE

"Share your knowledge. It is a way to achieve immortality."

Dalai Lama

It gives us great pleasure to write a Hand book of Ear, Nose, Throat and mouth disorders. This book is primarily intended for nursing students, the book particularly emphasizes on nursing care in ENT disorders and mouth disorders, realizing that nursing students are under increasing pressure to study more these days. which is important for nursing students, as they have to take both theory and clinical.

We hope that this book will also serve as a   reference book to GNMS and under graduate nursing students.

Vijayabarathi. M

S. Pauline Sheela Priya

J. Regina Margret Vimala

ACKNOWLEDGMENTS

First and fore most we wish to express our heartfelt thanks to all the contributors who have shown a steady faith in completion of this book.

We owe an undividable gratitude to god almighty for showing his immense grace upon us to carry out this book.

Thanks is such a small word but it contains a heartful of gratitude. The gratitude expressed is not a result of formality but is birthed from within. It is an appreciation to all those who motivated, guided and encouraged us throughout my study and stay here.

We are privileged to express our sincere thanks and gratitude to Dr. V. Hemavathy, MSc(N), M.A, M. Phil, Ph.D., Principal, Sree Balaji College of Nursing, Chrompet, Chennai, for guiding us to uplift our professional career by her valuable and constant guidance.

We are very much grateful to our beloved parents and family members, for their support, constant encouragement, inspiration which boosted up our morale during this work.

INDEX

INTRODUCTION

Some problems of the ear, nose and throat (ENT) are very common; most people at some time in their lives suffer from nosebleeds, sore throats or earache. Many of these problems will be dealt with successfully at home, often with the advice of a pharmacist or general practitioner (GP). Some ENT problems, however, can be life threatening, requiring an immediate visit to an emergency department (ED), surgery and, in some cases, a period of nursing care at home following discharge.

To nurse ENT patients effectively in a home or hospital setting, a basic knowledge of the anatomy and physiology of the relevant structures, along with a thorough understanding of the clinical features of common disorders, is essential. The health visitor, community nurse, school nurse or occupational health nurse is often in a position to detect problems before the medical practitioner or even the patient is aware of them.

This chapter will outline the basic structure and functioning of the ear, nose and throat, describing the most commonly encountered disorders of each, and outlining appropriate medical and nursing interventions. As in every area of nursing care, one of the most important contributions that nurses can make is in the area of communication and education as they provide support and reassurance to the patient and family, and convey information about the causes of the patient's condition, its treatment and measures to prevent its recurrence.

CHAPTER 1

REVIEW OF ANATOMY AND PHYSIOLOGY OF EAR, NOSE, THROAT

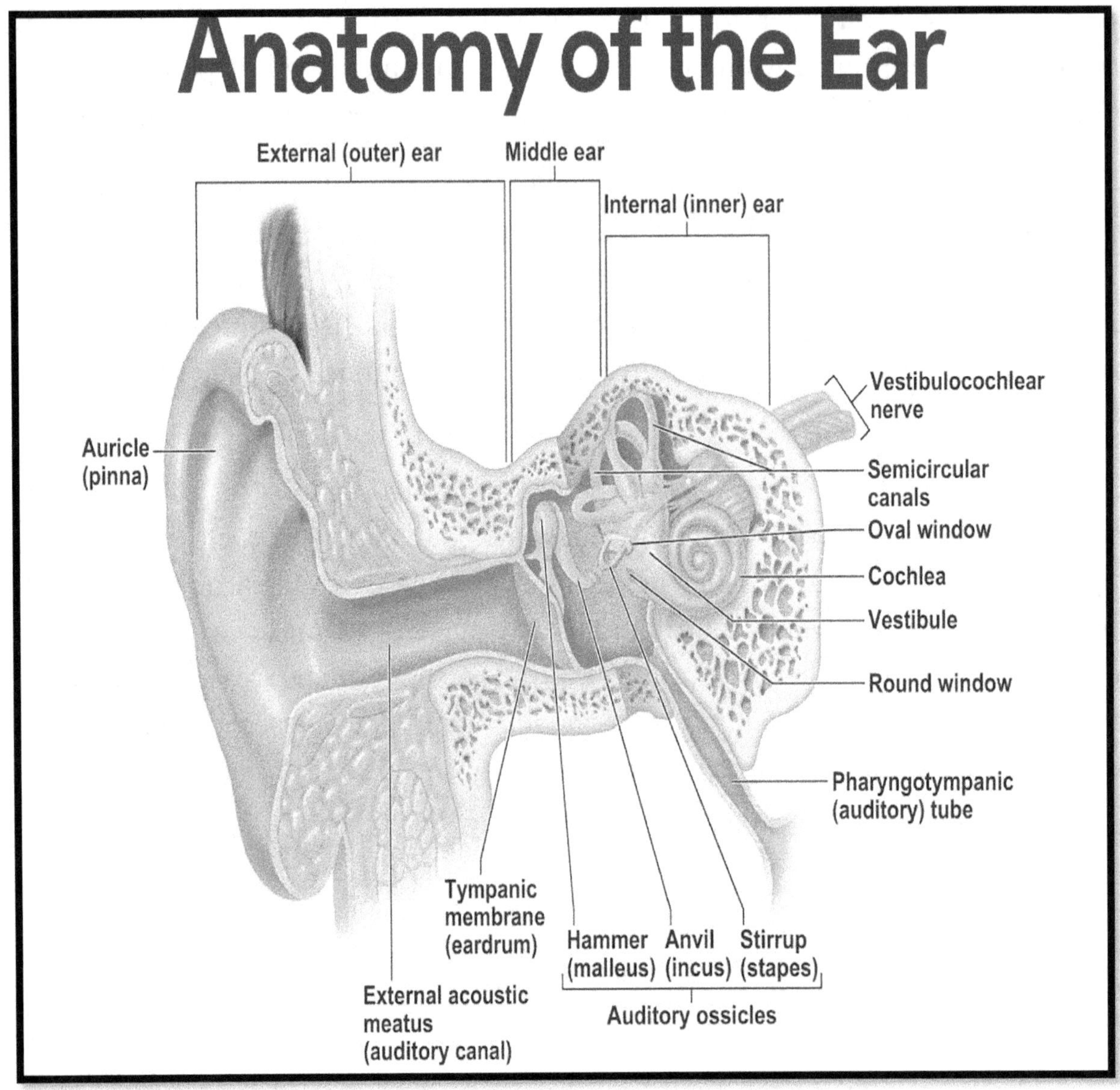

THE EAR: HEARING AND BALANCE

Anatomy of the Ear

Anatomically, the ear is divided into three major areas: the external, or outer ear the middle ear, and the internal, or inner, ear.

External (Outer) Ear

The external, or outer, ear is composed of the auricle and the external acoustic meatus.

Auricle. The auricle, or pinna, is what most people call the "ear"- the shell-shaped structure surrounding the auditory canal opening.

External acoustic meatus. The external acoustic meatus is a short, narrow chamber carved into the temporal bone of the skull; in its skin-lined walls are the ceruminous glands, which secrete waxy, yellow cerumen or earwax, which provides a sticky trap for foreign bodies and repels insects.

Tympanic membrane. Sound waves entering the auditory canal eventually hit the tympanic membrane, or eardrum, and cause it to vibrate; the canal ends at the ear drum, which separates the external from the middle ear.

Middle Ear

The middle ear, or tympanic cavity, is a small, air-filled, mucosa-lined cavity within the temporal bone.

Openings. The tympanic cavity is flanked laterally by the eardrum and medially by a bony wall with two openings, the oval window and the inferior, membrane-covered round window.

Pharyngotympanic tube. The pharyngotympanic tube runs obliquely downward to link the middle ear cavity with the throat, and the mucosae lining the two regions are continuous.

Ossicles. The tympanic cavity is spanned by the three smallest bones in the body, the ossicles, which transmit the vibratory motion of the eardrum to the fluids of the inner ear; these bones, named for their shape, are the hammer, or malleus, the anvil, or incus, and the stirrup, or stapes.

Internal (Inner) Ear

The internal ear is a maze of bony chambers, called the bony, or osseous, labyrinth, located deep within the temporal bone behind the eye socket.

Subdivisions. The three subdivisions of the bony labyrinth are the spiraling, pea-sized cochlea, the vestibule, and the semicircular canals.

Perilymph. The bony labyrinth is filled with a plasma-like fluid called perilymph.

Membranous labyrinth. Suspended in the perilymph is a membranous labyrinth, a system of membrane sacs that more or less follows the shape of the bony labyrinth.

Endolymph. The membranous labyrinth itself contains a thicker fluid called endolymph.

Chemical Senses: Taste and Smell

The receptors for taste and olfaction are classified as chemoreceptors because they respond to chemicals in solution.

Olfactory Receptors and the Sense of Smell

Even though our sense of smell is far less acute than that of many other animals, the human nose is still no slouch in picking up small differences in odours.

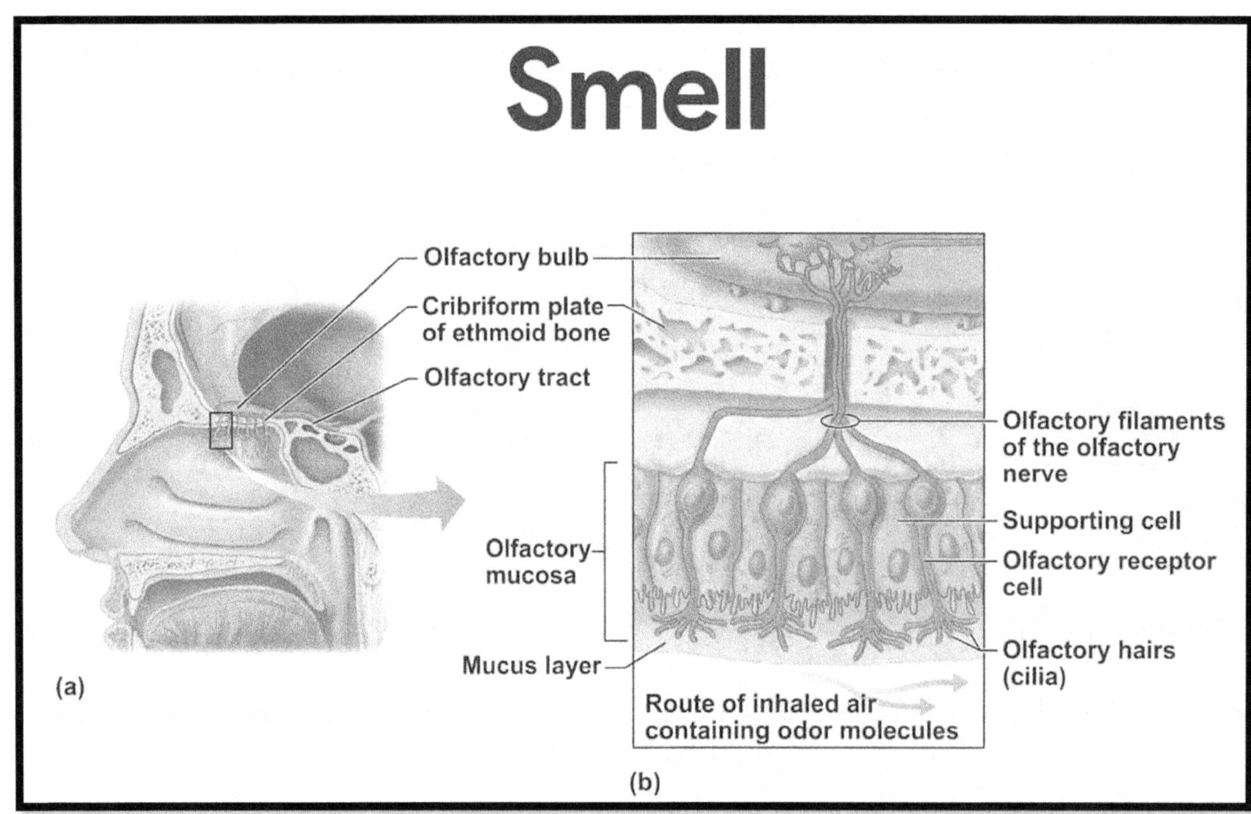

Olfactory receptors. The thousands of olfactory receptors, receptors for the sense of smell, occupy a postage stamp-sized area in the roof of each nasal cavity.

Olfactory receptor cells. The olfactory receptor cells are neurons equipped with olfactory hairs, long cilia that protrude from the nasal epithelium and are continuously bathed by a layer of mucus secreted by underlying glands.

Olfactory filaments. When the olfactory receptors located on the cilia are stimulated by chemicals dissolved in the mucus, they transmit impulses along the olfactory filaments, which are bundled axons of olfactory neurons that collectively make up the olfactory nerve.

Olfactory nerve. The olfactory nerve conducts the impulses to the olfactory cortex of the brain.

Taste Buds and the Sense of Taste

The word taste comes from the Latin word tax are, which means "to touch, estimate, or judge".

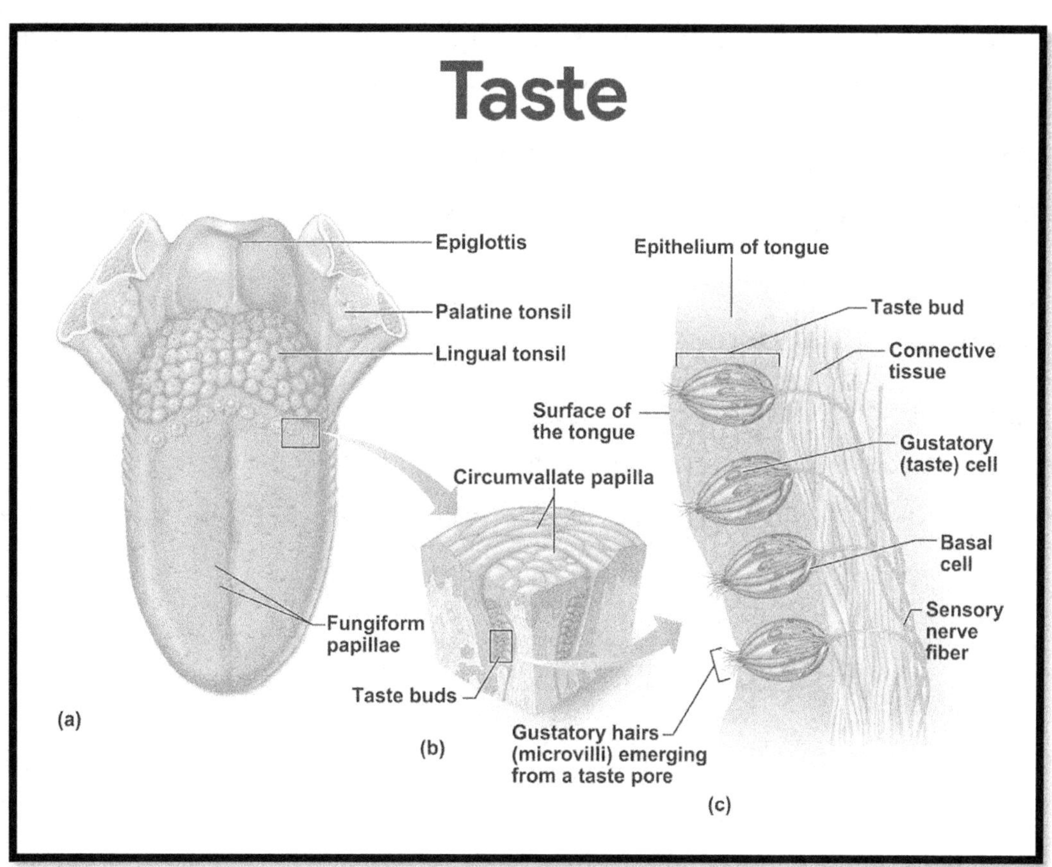

Taste buds. The taste buds, or specific receptors for the sense of taste, are widely scattered in the oral cavity; of the 10, 000 or so taste buds we have, most are on the tongue.

Papillae. The dorsal tongue surface is covered with small peg-like projections, or papillae.

Circumvallate and fungiform papillae. The taste buds are found on the sides of the large round circumvallate papillae and on the tops of the more numerous fungiform papillae.

Gustatory cells. The specific cells that respond to chemicals dissolved in the saliva are epithelial cells called gustatory cells.

Gustatory hairs. Their long microvilli- the gustatory hairs- protrude through the taste pore, and when they are stimulated, they depolarize and impulses are transmitted to the brain.

Facial nerve. The facial nerve (VII) serves the anterior part of the tongue.

Glossopharyngeal and vagus nerves. The other two cranial nerves- the glossopharyngeal and vagus- serve the other taste bud-containing areas.

Basal cells. Taste bud cells are among the most dynamic cells in the body, and they are replaced every seven to ten days by basal cells found in the deeper regions of the taste buds.

Mechanisms of Equilibrium

The equilibrium receptors of the inner ear, collectively called the vestibular apparatus, can be divided into two functional arms- one arm responsible for monitoring static equilibrium and the other involved with dynamic equilibrium.

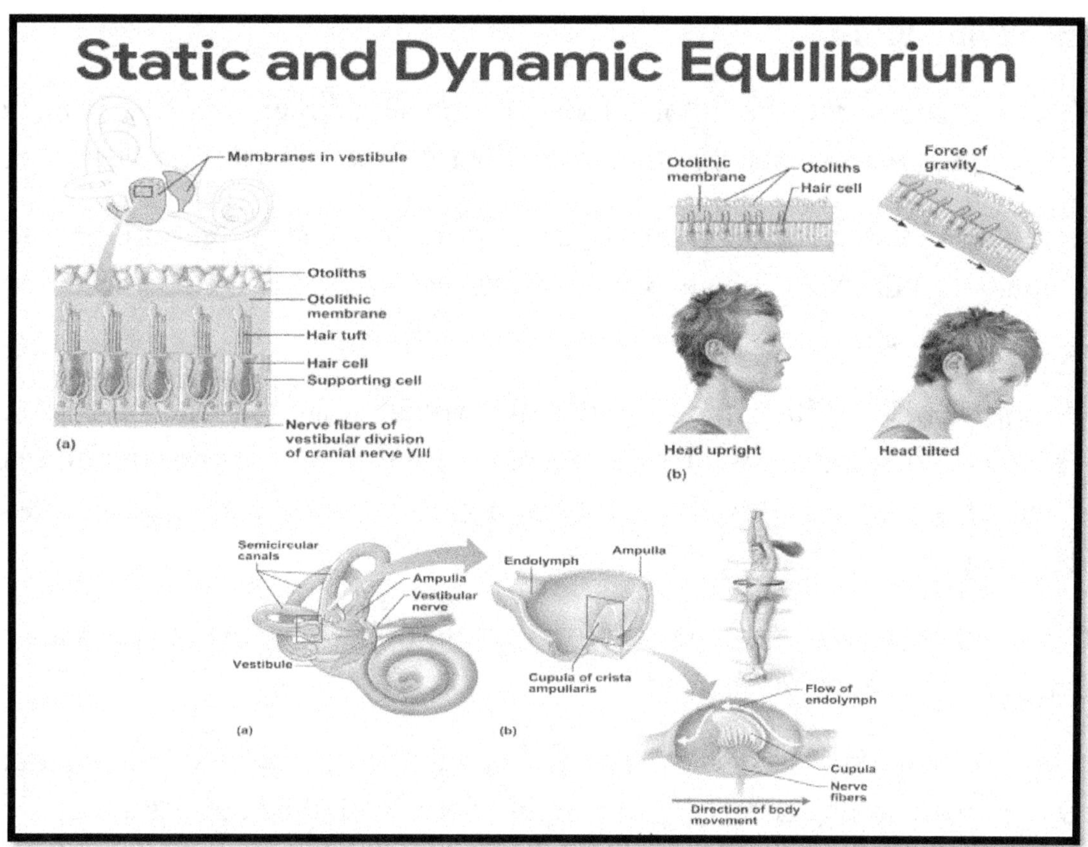

Static Equilibrium

Within the membrane sacs of the vestibule are receptors called maculae that are essential to our sense of static equilibrium.

Maculae. The maculae report on changes in the position of the head in space with respect to the pull of gravity when the body is not moving.

Otolithic hair membrane. Each macula is a patch of receptor (hair) cells with their "hairs" embedded in the otolithic hair membrane, a jelly-like mass studded with otoliths, tiny stones made of calcium salts.

Otoliths. As the head moves, the otoliths roll in response to changes in the pull of gravity; this movement creates a pull on the gel, which in turn slides like a greased plate over the hair cells, bending their hairs.

Vestibular nerve. This event activates the hair cells, which send impulses along the vestibular nerve (a division of cranial nerve VIII) to the cerebellum of the brain, informing it of the position of the head in space.

Dynamic Equilibrium

The dynamic equilibrium receptors, found in the semicircular canals, respond to angular or rotatory movements of the head rather than to straight-line movements.

Semicircular canals. The semicircular canals are oriented in the three planes of space; thus regardless of which plane one moves in, there will be receptors to detect the movement.

Crista ampullaris. Within the ampulla, a swollen region at the base of each membranous semicircular canal is a receptor region called crista ampullaris, or simply crista, which consists of a tuft of hair cells covered with a gelatinous cap called the cupula.

Head movements. When the head moves in an arclike or angular direction, the endolymph in the canal lags behind.

Bending of the cupula. Then, as the cupula drags against the stationary endolymph, the cupula bends- like a swinging door- with the body's motion.

Vestibular nerve. This stimulates the hair cells, and impulses are transmitted up the vestibular nerve to the cerebellum.

Mechanism of Hearing

The following is the route of sound waves through the ear and activation of the cochlear hair cells.

Vibrations. To excite the hair cells in the organ of Corti in the inner ear, sound wave vibrations must pass through air, membranes, bone and fluid.

Sound transmission. The cochlea is drawn as though it were uncoiled to make the events of sound transmission occurring there easier to follow.

Low frequency sound waves. Sound waves of low frequency that are below the level of hearing travel entirely around the cochlear duct without exciting hair cells.

High frequency sound waves. But sounds of higher frequency result in pressure waves that penetrate through the cochlear duct and basilar membrane to reach the scala tympani; this causes the basilar membrane to vibrate maximally in certain areas in response to certain frequencies of sound, stimulating particular hair cells and sensory neurons.

Length of fibers. The length of the fibers spanning the basilar membrane tune specific regions to vibrate at specific frequencies; the higher notes- 20, 000 Hertz (Hz)- are detected by shorter hair cells along the base of the basilar membrane.

The Nose

The nose is the only externally visible part of the respiratory system.

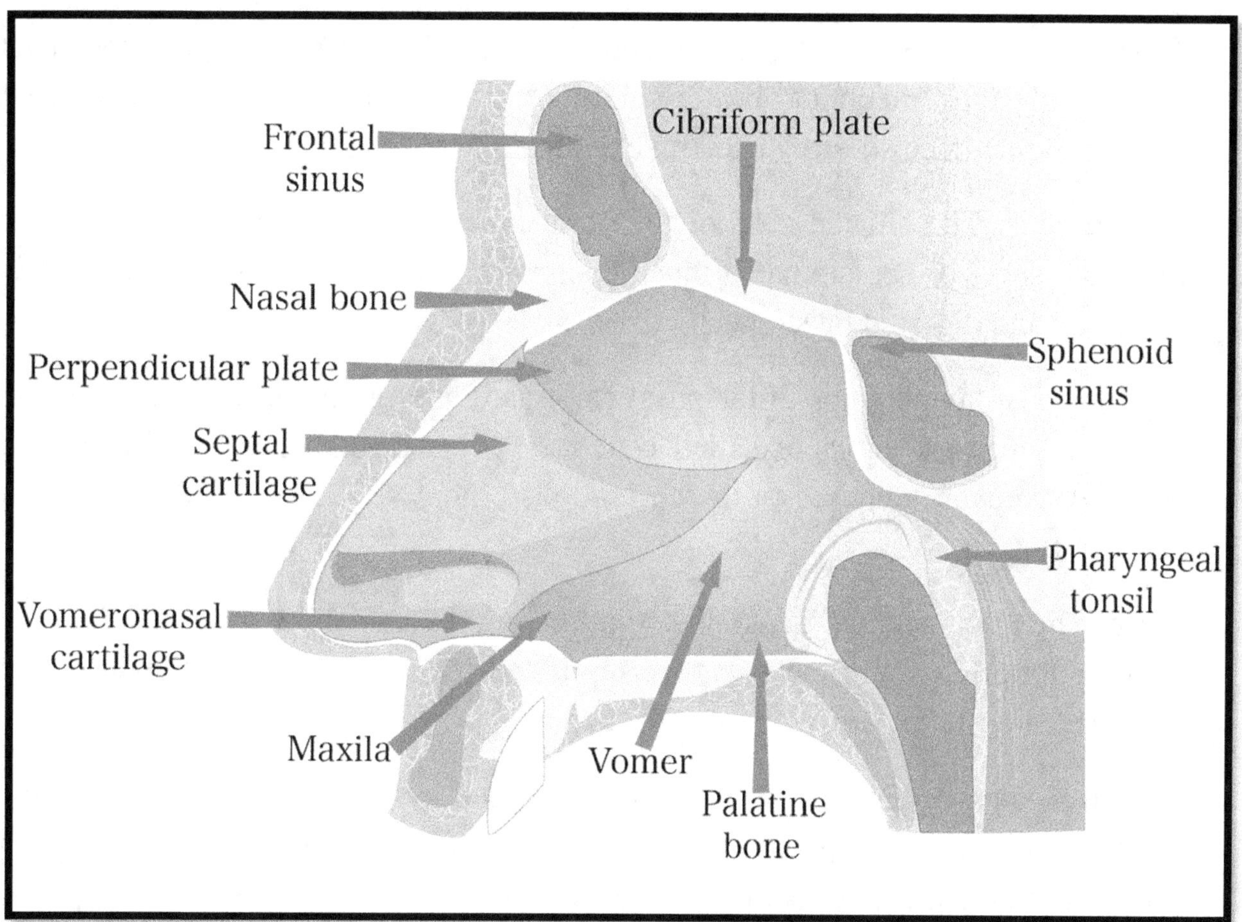

Nostrils. During breathing, air enters the nose by passing through the nostrils, or nares.

Nasal cavity. The interior of the nose consists of the nasal cavity, divided by a midline nasal septum.

Olfactory receptors. The olfactory receptors for the sense of smell are located in the mucosa in the slit like superior part of the nasal cavity, just beneath the ethmoid bone.

Respiratory mucosa. The rest of the mucosal lining, the nasal cavity called the respiratory mucosa, rests on a rich network of thin-walled veins that warms the air as it flows past.

Mucus. In addition, the sticky mucus produced by the mucosa's glands moistens the air and traps incoming bacteria and other foreign debris, and lysozyme enzymes in the mucus destroy bacteria chemically.

Ciliated cells. The ciliated cells of the nasal mucosa create a gentle current that moves the sheet of contaminated mucus posteriorly toward the throat, where it is swallowed and digested by stomach juices.

Conchae. The lateral walls of the nasal cavity are uneven owing to three mucosa-covered projections, or lobes called conchae, which greatly increase the surface area of the mucosa exposed to the air, and also increase the air turbulence in the nasal cavity.

Palate. The nasal cavity is separated from the oral cavity below by a partition, the palate; anteriorly, where the palate is supported by bone, is the hard palate; the unsupported posterior part is the soft palate.

Paranasal sinuses. The nasal cavity is surrounded by a ring of paranasal sinuses located in the frontal, sphenoid, ethmoid, and maxillary bones; theses sinuses lighten the skull, and they act as a resonance chamber for speech.

Pharynx

Nose and pharynx anatomy

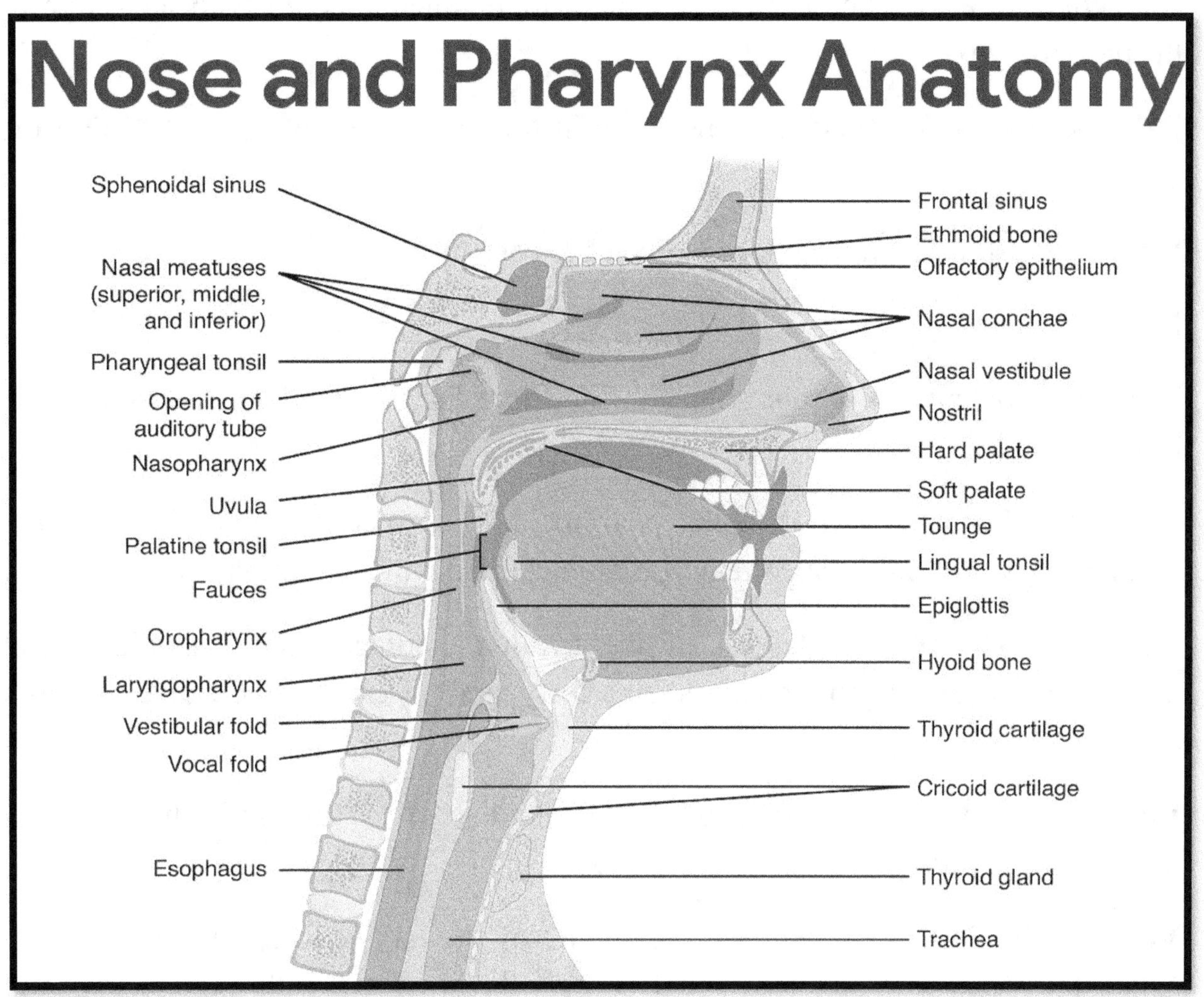

Size. The pharynx is a muscular passageway about 13 cm (5 inches) long that vaguely resembles a short length of red garden hose.

Function. Commonly called the throat, the pharynx serves as a common passageway for food and air.

Portions of the pharynx. Air enters the superior portion, the nasopharynx, from the nasal cavity and then descends through the oropharynx and laryngopharynx to enter the larynx below.

Pharyngotympanic tube. The pharyngotympanic tubes, which drain the middle ear open into the nasopharynx.

Pharyngeal tonsil. The pharyngeal tonsil, often called adenoid is located high in the nasopharynx.

Palatine tonsils. The palatine tonsils are in the oropharynx at the end of the soft palate.

Lingual tonsils. The lingual tonsils lie at the base of the tongue.

Larynx

The larynx or voice box routes air and food into the proper channels and plays a role in speech.

Structure. Located inferior to the pharynx, it is formed by eight rigid hyaline cartilages and a spoon-shaped flap of elastic cartilage, the epiglottis.

Thyroid cartilage. The largest of the hyaline cartilages is the shield-shaped thyroid cartilage, which protrudes anteriorly and is commonly called Adam's apple.

Epiglottis. Sometimes referred to as the "guardian of the airways", the epiglottis protects the superior opening of the larynx.

Vocal folds. Part of the mucous membrane of the larynx forms a pair of folds, called the vocal folds, or true vocal cords, which vibrate with expelled air and allows us to speak.

Glottis. The slitlike passageway between the vocal folds is the glottis.

Trachea

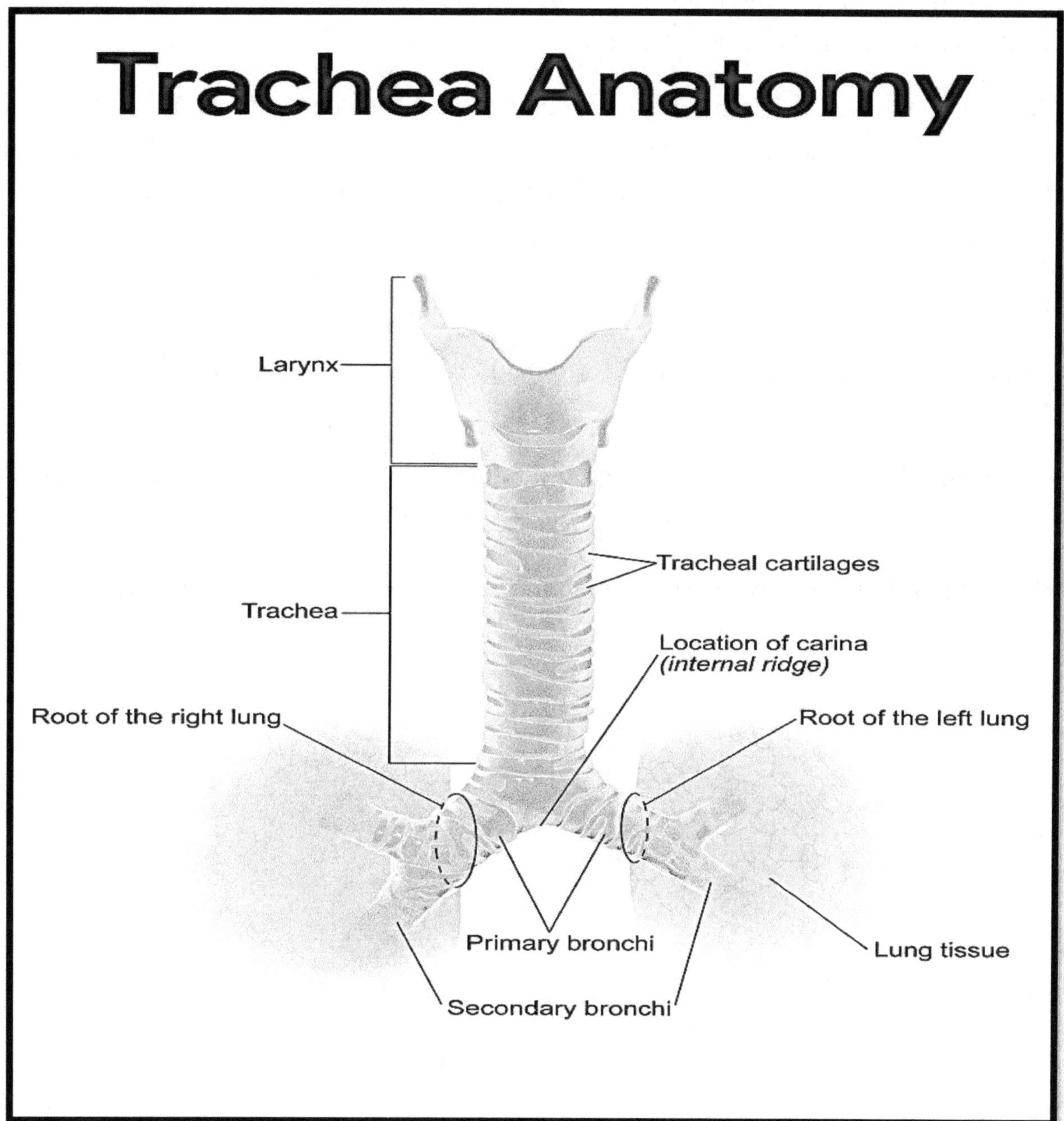

Length. Air entering the trachea or windpipe from the larynx travels down its length (10 to 12 cm or about 4 inches) to the level of the fifth thoracic vertebra, which is approximately mid chest.

Structure. The trachea is fairly rigid because its walls are reinforced with C-shaped rings of hyaline cartilage; the open parts of the rings about the oesophagus and allow it to expand anteriorly when we swallow a large piece of food, while the solid portions support the trachea walls and keep it patent, or open, in spite of the pressure changes that occur during breathing.

Cilia. The trachea is lined with ciliated mucosa that beat continuously and in a direction opposite to that of the incoming air as they propel mucus, loaded with dust particles and other debris away from the lungs to the throat, where it can be swallowed or spat out.

Main Bronchi

Structure. The right and left main (primary) bronchi are formed by the division of the trachea.

Location. Each main bronchus runs obliquely before it plunges into the medial depression of the lung on its own side.

Size. The right main bronchus is wider, shorter, and straighter than the left.

CHAPTER - 2

ASSESSMENT OF THE EAR, NOSE, THROAT

History:

The following issues should be included:

- Classic symptoms of ear disease: deafness, tinnitus, discharge (otorrhoea), pain (otalgia) and vertigo.
- Previous ear surgery, or head injury.
- Family history of deafness.
- Systemic disease (eg, stroke, multiple sclerosis, cardiovascular disease).
- Ototoxic drugs (antibiotics (eg, Gentamicin), diuretics, cyto toxics).
- Exposure to noise (eg, pneumatic drill or shooting).
- History of atopy and allergy in children.
- Inspecting the external ear
- Inspect the external ear before examination with an otoscope / auriscope. Swab any discharge and remove any wax. Look for obvious signs of abnormality.
- Size and shape of the pinna.
- Extra cartilage tags/pre-auricular sinuses or pits.
- Signs of trauma to the pinna.
- Suspicious skin lesions on the pinna, including neoplasia.
- Skin conditions of the pinna and external canal.
- Infection/inflammation of the external ear canal, with discharge.
- Signs/scars of previous surgery.
- Inspecting the ear canal and eardrum
- A modern electric otoscope /auriscope with its own light source is primarily used to examine the ear. An otoscope also has its own magnification, which gives a good view of the tympanic membrane (TM). Batteries need to be fully operational to allow optimal light during examination.

The examination technique involves grasping the pinna and pulling it up and backwards (posteriorly and superiorly), which helps to straighten the ear canal and for inspection of the TM. (In infants, only pull the pinna posteriorly not superiorly for examination.)

Hold the otoscope near to the eyepiece rather than at the end; this helps to reduce the patient's discomfort due to hand movements, which are exaggerated in the ear. Modern otoscopes are designed to use a disposable speculum. It is necessary to fit the correct size of speculum to achieve the best view; it is tempting to use a small piece for ease of insertion, but this simply restricts the image available.

Note the condition of the canal skin, and the presence of wax, foreign tissue, or discharge. The mobility of the eardrum can be evaluated using a pneumatic speculum, which attaches to the otoscope. The drum should move on squeezing the balloon.

Inspecting the tympanic membrane

Move the otoscope in order to see several different views of the drum; it is not always possible to see the whole drum in one single view using an otoscope. The drum is roughly circular (~ 1 cm in diameter). In a normal drum the following structures can be identified:

- Handle/lateral process of the malleus.
- Light reflex/cone of light.
- Pars tensa and pars flaccida (attic).

Occasionally, in a healthy, thin drum, it is possible to see the following:

- Long process of incus.
- Chorda tympani.
- Eustachian opening.
- Promontory of the cochlea.

Common pathological conditions related to the ear include:

- Perforations (note size, site and position).
- Tympanosclerosis.
- Glue ear/middle-ear effusion.

- Retractions of the drum.
- Haemo tympanum (blood in the middle ear).
- Check facial nerve function if ear pathology is serious.

Basic hearing tests

Detailed hearing tests are usually performed in audiology clinics.

A patient with normal hearing should hear equally as well in both ears.

Tuning fork tests: Weber's test and Rinne's test:

Weber's test - this is performed in conjunction with Rinne's test. The vibrating fork is placed in the middle of the forehead and the patient is asked whether any sound is heard and, if so, whether it is equally heard in both ears or not. In a patient with normal hearing, the tone is heard centrally. If the patient has unilateral hearing loss and the sound is louder in the weaker ear, this suggests a conductive hearing loss. If the sound is louder in the better ear, it is more likely to be a sensorineural hearing loss.

Rinne's test - strike a tuning fork and hold it vertically with its nearest prong about 1 cm away from the patient's external auditory meatus, making sure that it is not touching any hair. Then immediately transfer it to the mastoid process and hold it firmly there (applying counter pressure to the opposite side of the head) for two seconds. The patient is asked to report on which of the two positions was the louder. Normally, the patient should hear the air conduction better than the bone conduction (ie first position better than the second). This is a positive Rinne's test. If the Rinne's test is positive and there is hearing impairment, it is a sensorineural and not a conductive problem. If there is a negative Rinne's test with hearing loss, then the problem is a conductive one.

Free field voice testing (whisper from 40 cm)

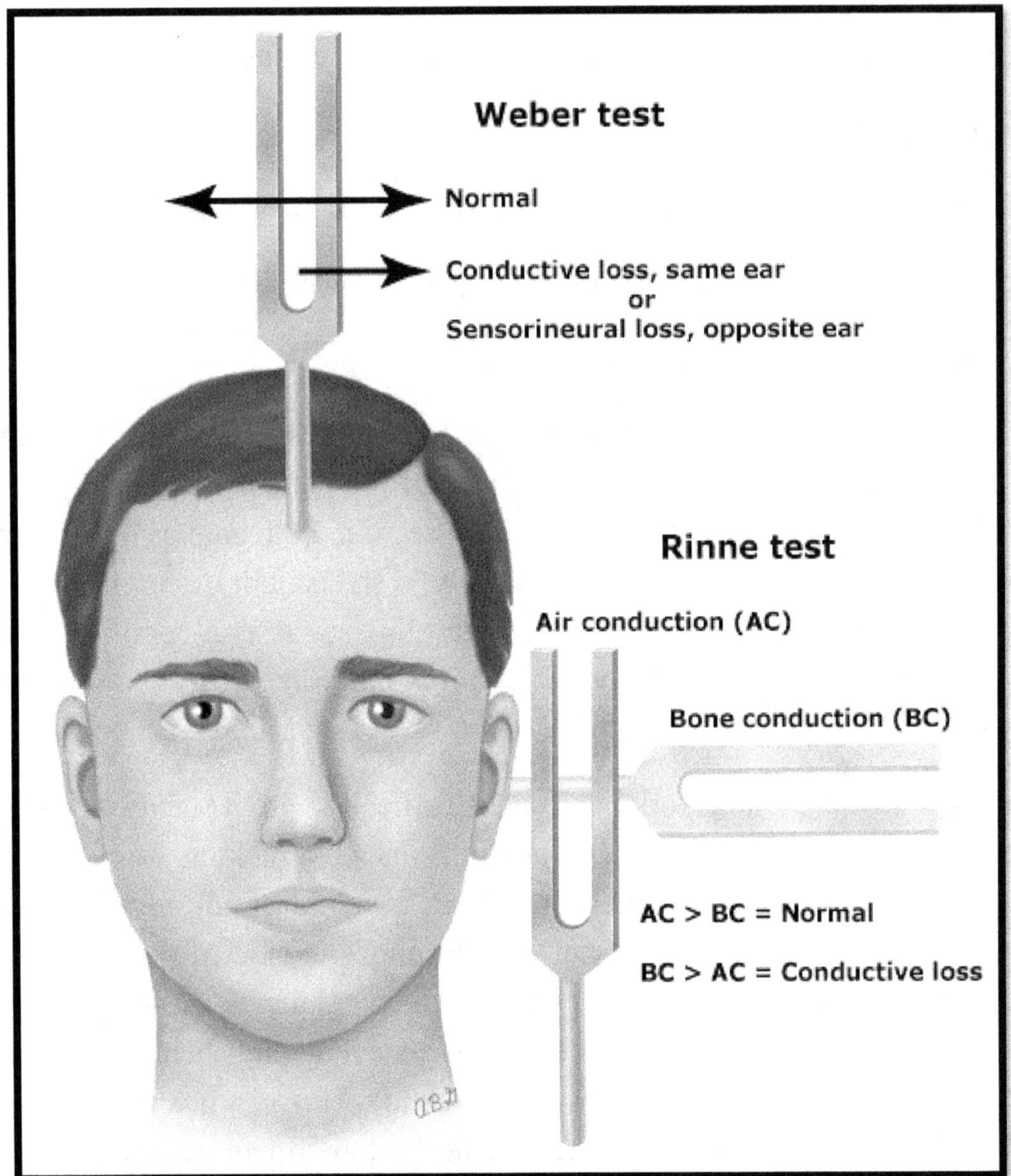

Examination of the nose

Full nose examinations assess the function, airway resistance and occasionally sense of smell. It includes looking into the mouth and pharynx. Common symptoms of nasal disease include:

- Airway obstruction.
- Rhinorrhoea (runny nose).
- Sneezing.

- Loss of smell (anosmia).
- Facial pain caused by sinusitis.
- Snoring (associated with nasal obstruction).

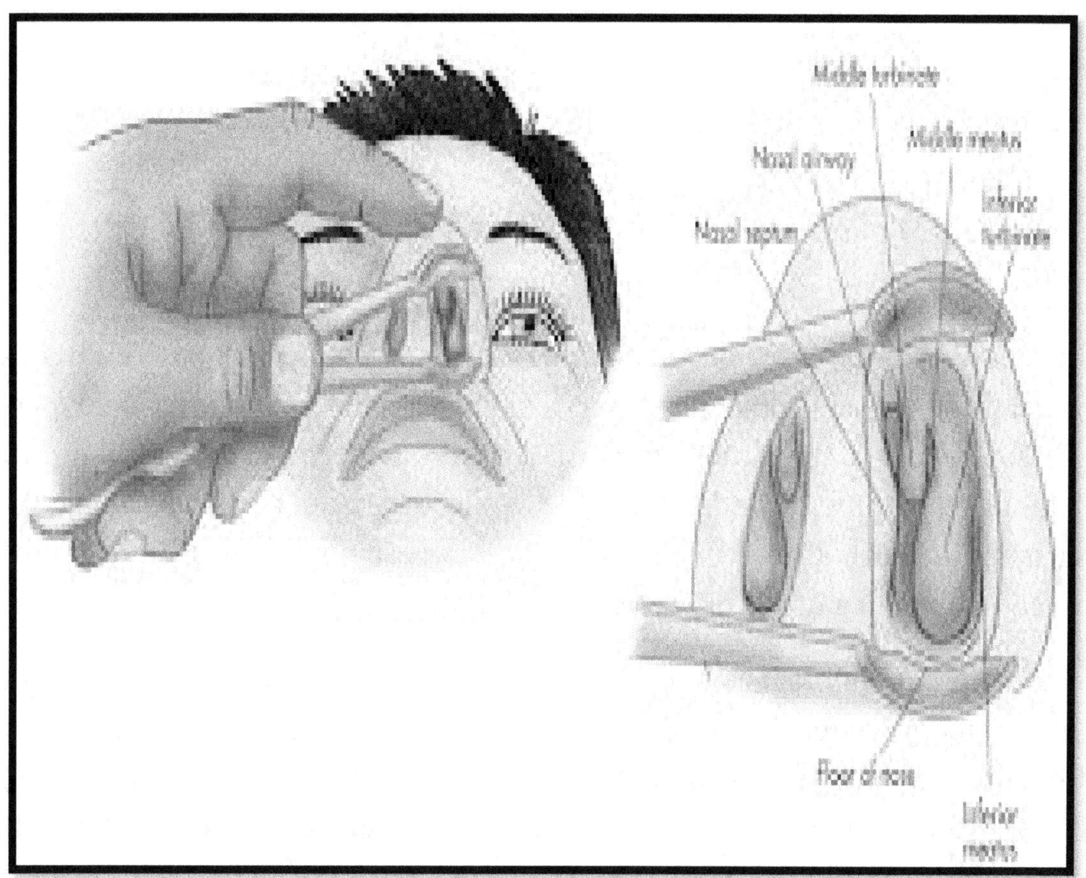

History

The following issues should be covered:

- Allergies/atopic disease.
- Smoking.
- Pets at home.
- Occupation.
- History of previous surgery.
- Previous trauma.
- General medical history.
- Seasonal or daily variation in symptoms.
- Inspection of the nose

- First look at the external nose. Ask the patient to remove any glasses. Look at the nose from the front and side for any signs of the following:
- Size and shape.
- Obvious bend or deformity: a deviated nose is often best looked at from above.
- Swelling.
- Scars or abnormal creases.
- Redness (evidence of skin disease).
- Discharge or crusting.
- Offensive smell.

The nose can be inspected from the front to examine the anterior nares by lifting the tip of the nose up and looking inside without a speculum. Check patency of each side and ask the patient to sniff. To assess the nasal airway hold a cold metal tongue compressor under the nose while the patient exhales and note the condensation under both nostrils, or occlude one nostril whilst the patient sniffs to give a reasonable idea of airway patency.

Most otolaryngologists use either a head mirror or illuminated spectacles with a Thudichum speculum to open up the nose, which allows examination of the nasal cavity. Holding the instrument comfortably can take practice at first. Insert the Thudichum speculum gently, and identify the nasal septum medially; turbines laterally; inferior turbinate (nearly always possible to see); the middle turbinate is often difficult to see as it is small.

Check for inflammation (rhinitis), position of the septum, and presence of polyps (touch to check sensitivity; it should be insensitive to touch). A foreign body, usually accompanied by an offensive unilateral discharge, may be seen inside the nose of a child.

A mirror and headlight or an endoscope instrument are used to view the nasopharynx (the postnasal space, which contains the Eustachian tube orifices and pharyngeal recess (of Rosenmüller) and may contain adenoids or nasopharyngeal cancer), but this is not always possible during a routine examination. Finally, examine the palate. Look for large nasal polyps and tumours arising from the soft palate.

Examination of the throat

This includes a thorough examination of the oral cavity.

History

General history, plus ask the patient about tobacco or alcohol use and dental history.

Inspection

Ask the patient to remove dentures, and examine their mouth systemically (use a bright torch): tongue, hard and soft palate, tonsillar fossa, gingivolabial/gingivobuccal sulci, floor of mouth/under surface of tongue as follows:

Examine the mouth and note the condition of the tongue.

- Examine back of tongue and tonsils (press down on the tongue with a tongue depressor).
- Palpate the base of the tongue (look for tumours that may not be easily visible).
- Inspect the uvula and soft palate.
- Inspect the hard palate (ask the patient to tip their head backwards, until the whole hard palate is visible).
- Examine the buccal area and the gingivolabial (gingiva buccal) sulcus (the space between cheek and gums).
- Examine the floor of the mouth, check for submandibular duct stones or masses (ask the patient to stick their tongue out).
- Examine the naso pharynx and larynx with a mirror or flexible fibreoptic naso endoscope.

DIAGNOSTIC PROCEDURES IN DISORDERS OF THE EAR

Inspection and palpation of the pinna.

Otoscopy: Inspection of the external auditory meatus and tympanic membrane with an otoscope, an instrument that directs light into the ear through a conical speculum, and is equipped with a magnifying lens; mobility of the tympanic membrane can be assessed when the subject swallows or performs the Valsalva maneuver (or when, in children, the examiner blows a puff of air into the ear with a rubber bulb attached to the otoscope).

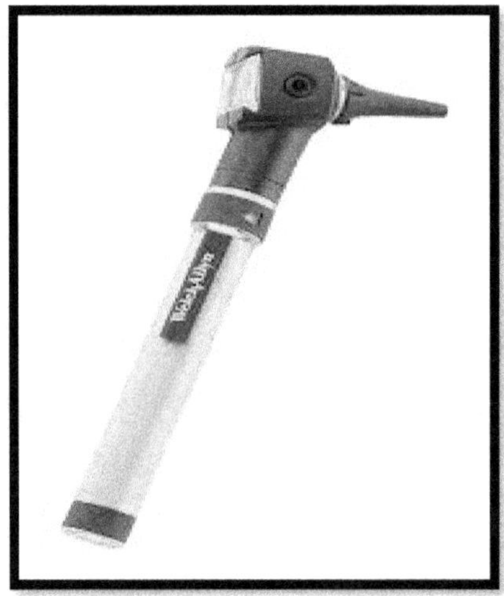

Measurements of hearing:

(1) simple tests with ticking watch or tuning fork;

(2) Audiography, a precise measurement of the faintest loudness (in decibels) that the subject can hear, each being ear tested separately at each of several pitches (for example,250, 500, 1000, 2000, 3000, 4000, 6000, and 8000Hz); this can be performed by a technician with carefully calibrated testing equipment, or by automated machinery activated by the subject;

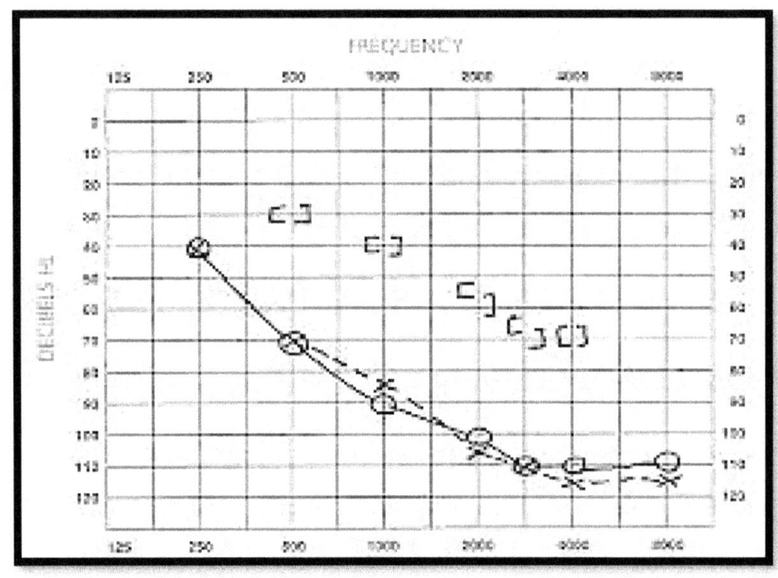

(3) more elaborate testing of the subject's ability to discriminate spoken words.

Weber test: A vibrating tuning fork placed firmly against a bony surface of the head at the midline sends vibrations through the bones of the skull. These should be heard equally in the two ears; if there is hearing loss due to blockage of the external auditory meatus or to injury or disease of the middle ear, the tone of the fork will be heard louder in the affected ear; in hearing loss due to damage to the inner ear or acoustic nerve, however, the tone will be heard louder in the more normal ear.

Rinne test: The sound of a vibrating tuning fork positioned so that the tines are near the pinna (air conduction) should be heard by the subject even after the sound sensed when the shank of the tuning fork is placed on the mastoid process behind the ear(bone conduction) can no longer be heard; when bone conduction is heard longer than air conduction in an ear with reduced hearing, the hearing lossis due to obstruction of the meatus or disease of the middle ear.

Tympano centesis: Puncture of the tympanic membrane and withdrawal of fluid from the middle ear for examination, including culture.

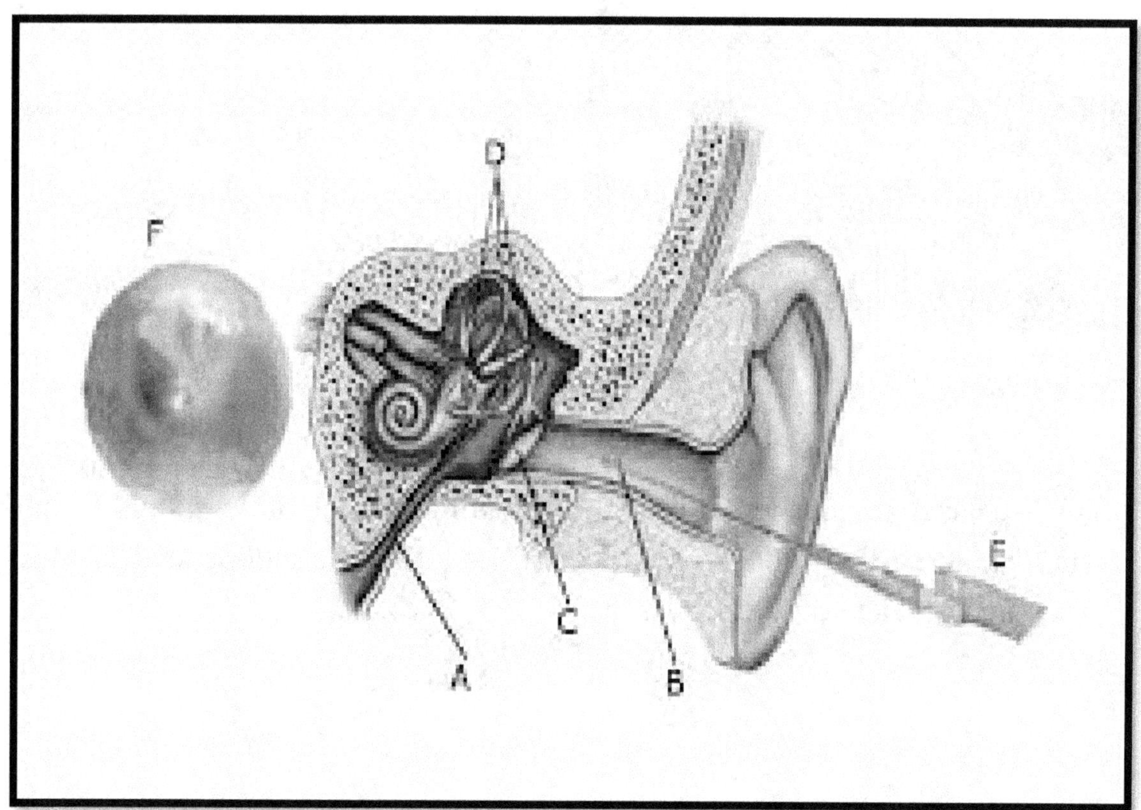

Pneumo tympanometry: Assessment of the mobility of the tympanic membrane by applying pressure to its outer surface with a device fitting tightly in the external meatus.

DIAGNOSTIC PROCEDURE IN DISORDERS OF THE NOSE

- Direct inspection with nasal speculum or rhinoscope.
- Posterior rhinoscopy: Inspection of posterior nares with angled mirror placed in the oropharynx.

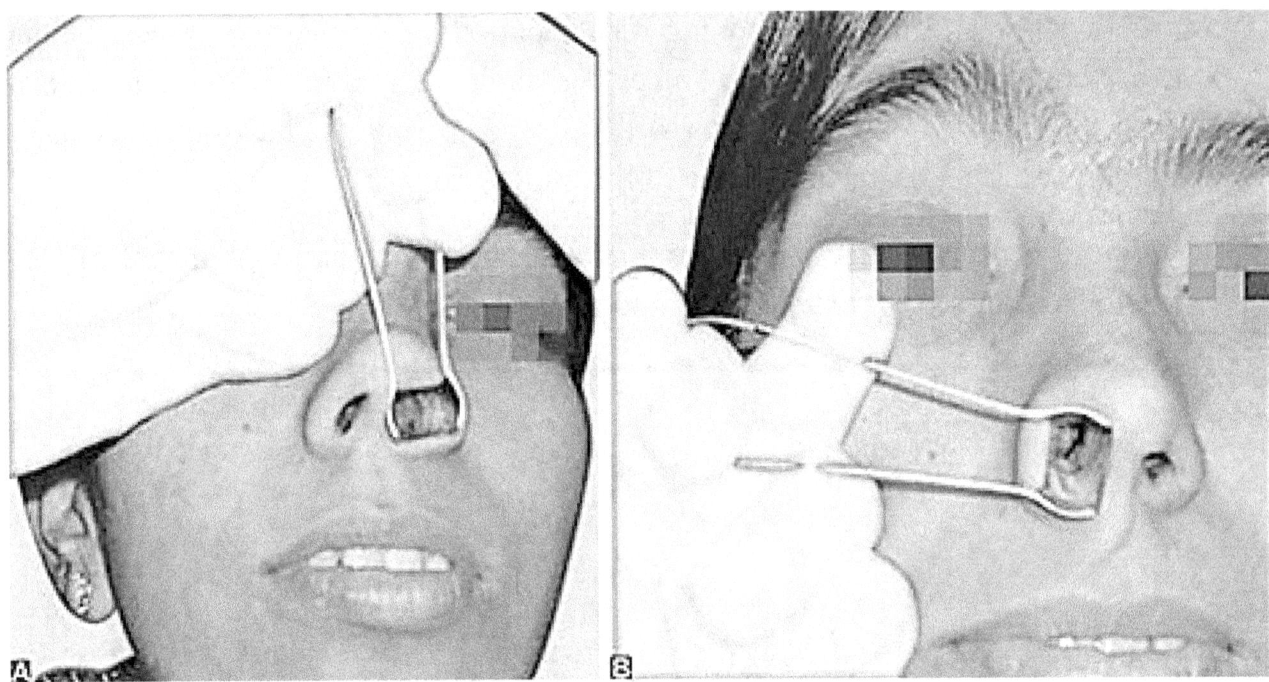

- **Nasal smear:** Examination of a stained smear of scrapings from the nasal mucosa for evidence of infection (neutrophilic leukocytes) or allergy (eosinophilic leukocytes).

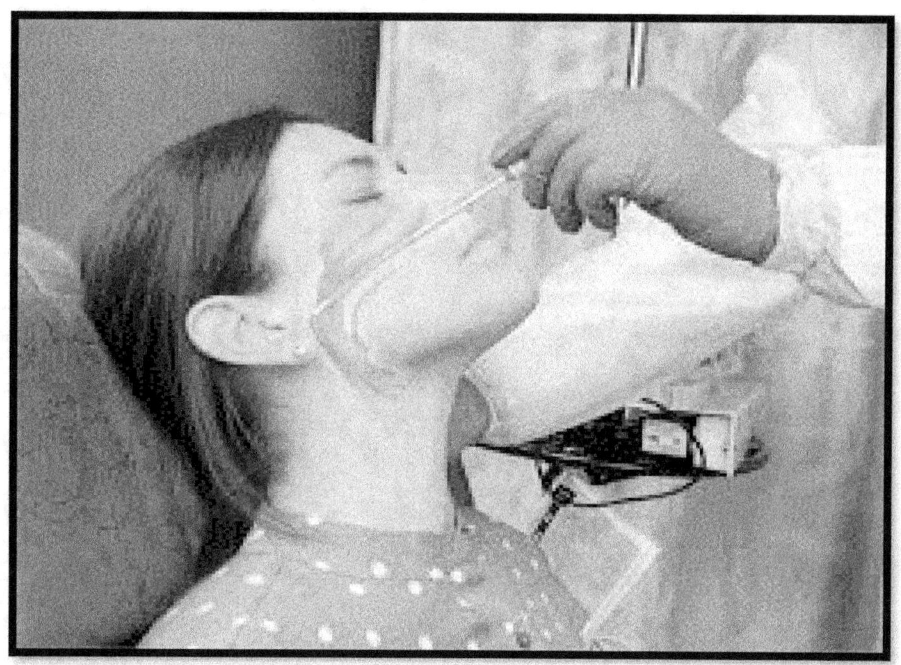

- Culture of nasal secretions to identify bacterial pathogens.

DIAGNOSTIC PROCEDURES IN DISORDERS OF THE THROAT

- Inspection of the throat with a focused light, often with the aid of a tongue depressor (tongue blade) to press the tongue out of the field of vision.

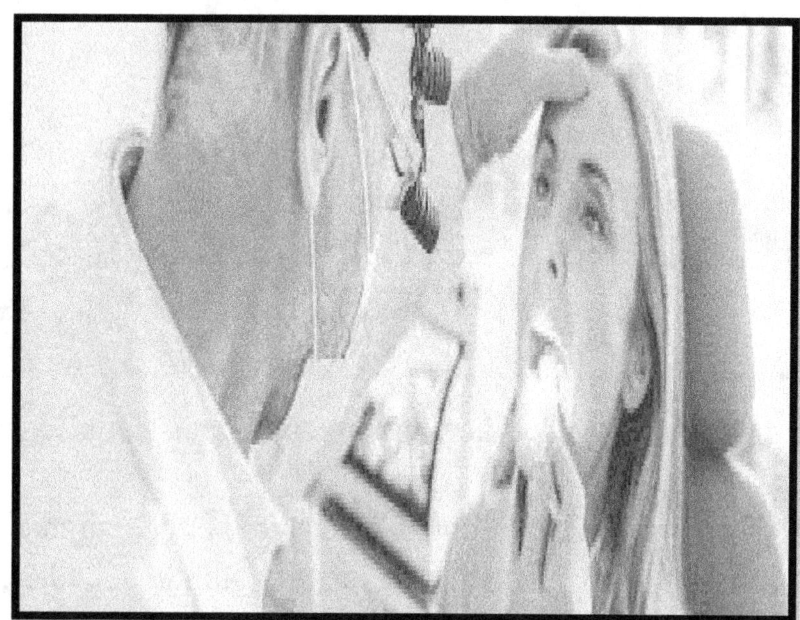

- Palpation of cervical lymph glands and of masses, swellings, or other structures within the throat.

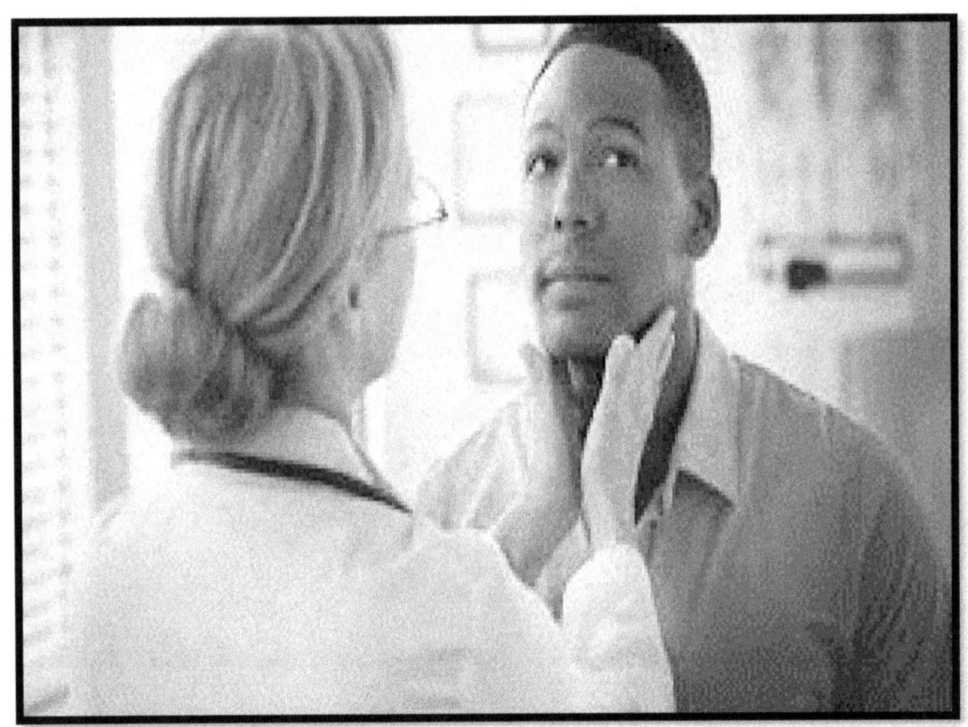

- Throat culture to identify bacterial pathogens.

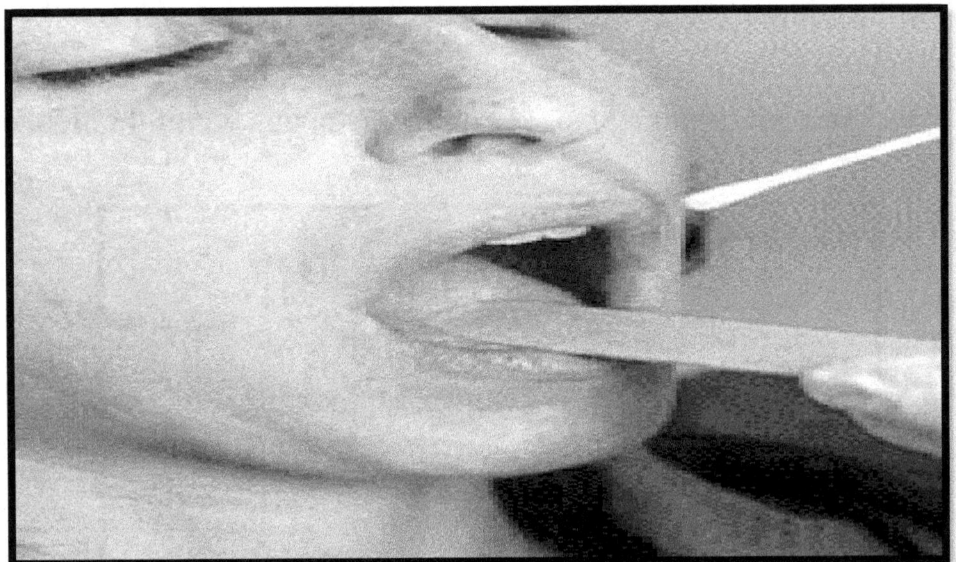

- Strep screen (faster than culture, but detects only group A beta-hemolytic streptococci).
- Biopsy of masses or lesions suspected of being malignant.
- X-ray or other imaging to identify foreign bodies, masses, or abnormalities of the airway due to injury or disease.

CHAPTER - 3

COMMON DISORDERS OF EAR, NOSE, THROAT

INFECTIONS OF THE OUTER AND MIDDLE EAR

Otitis Externa (Swimmer's Ear) : Infection of the external auditory meatus.

Causes: Infection with bacteria (Proteus, Pseudomonas) and sometimes fungi (Aspergillus). Predisposing causes include water exposure (swimming, showering), excessive cerumen, mechanical trauma(probing with paperclip), foreign body (cotton, pencil eraser), diabetes mellitus, and immune compromise.

Signs and symptoms : Earache, itching in the external auditory meatus, purulent discharge. Hearing loss if the meatus is occluded by swelling or exudate.

Physical Examination: Redness and swelling of the meatus, sometimes with complete occlusion; purulent exudate, perhaps with excessive cerumen or foreign body visible. Tenderness on manipulation of the pinna.

Course: Generally benign, but in diabetes mellitus and AIDS an external ear infection may resist conservative treatment and become chronic, perhaps

invading the skull or brain, with resulting neurologic damage.

Treatment: After gentle cleansing and removal of any foreign material, cerumen, or exudate, topical antibiotics (ear drops), often with hydrocortisone to combat local inflammation, are instilled several times a day. Sometimes a gauze wick is inserted to facilitate penetration of ear drops when edema of the meatus is extreme. In invasive infections, intravenous antibiotics and even surgery may be required.

Otitis Media

- It is the inflammation of the middle ear
- Bacterial infection of the middle ear and adjoining mastoid air cells.

Causes:

Organism responsible for Acute otitis media:

In children:
- Haemophilus influenza
- Streptococcus pneumonia
- Branhamella catarrhalis

In adults
- Staphylococcus aureus
- Beta haemolytic streptococcus
- Streptococcus pneumoniae

Chronic otitis media

Aerobes:
- Staphylococcus aureus
- Pseudomonasaeruginosa
- Streptococci
- Klebsiella
- Proteusspecies

Anaerobes:
- bacteroides

Otitis media is often bilateral. It is commoner in infants and small children than in adolescents and adults, accounting for one-third of all hospital visits.

Pathophysiology:

Viral/bacterial infection
⇓
Infection and inflammation
⇓
Otitis media
⇓
Recurrent infection
⇓
cholesteatoma

Signs and symptoms:

Acute otitis media

- Pain
- fever
- hearing loss

Active stage:

Ear discharge- moderate profuse, mucopurulent colorless greenish yellow.

Chronic:

- Hearing loss(conductive)
- Foul smelling otorrhea

Acute mastoiditis:

- Post auricular area tenderness
- Erythematous edematous
- Perforation of tympanic membrane (varying in size and shape)
- vertigo

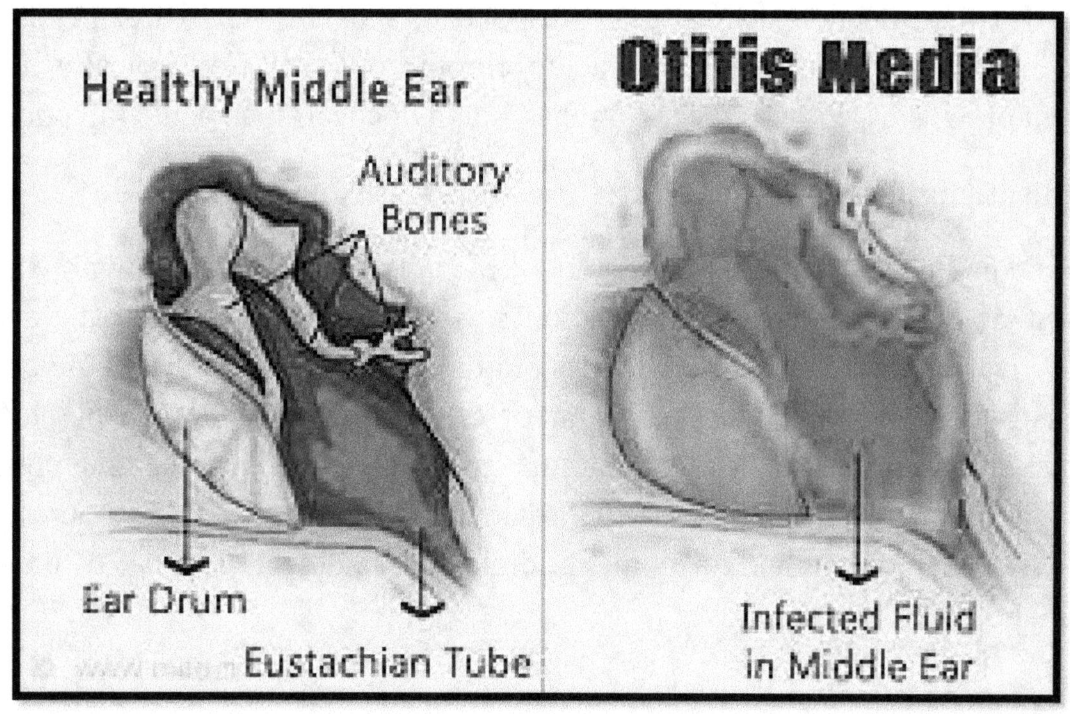

Diagnostic method:

- History collection
- physical examination
  Redness of the tympanic membrane, sometimes with formation of bullae. Immobility of the tympanic membrane, reflecting malfunction of the auditory tube. Occasionally bulging of the membrane. If spontaneous rupture occurs, blood or purulent exudate in the external auditory meatus.
- Otoscopy
- Audiogram
- Pus c/s
- Sinus x-ray
- x-ray mastoid
- MRI
- Ct scan of temporal bone

Course:

It is estimated that 20-80% of all cases of otitis media will resolve spontaneously without treatment. When there is fever or severe pain, antibiotic treatment is usually prescribed because of the risk of serious complications in a few patients. Neglect of the infection, its failure to respond to standard initial treatment, or a series of recurrent infections can lead to chronic otitis media, typically due to different organisms (Proteus, Pseudomonas, staphylococci) than acute infection.

Complications of chronic otitis

media include spontaneous rupture of the tympanic membrane, with chronic purulent drainage; destruction of the bones within the middle ear that transmit sound; invasion of mastoid air cells (mastoiditis), skull bones, and even the central nervous system by infection; formation of cholesteatoma, a benign but locally invasive growth of the tympanic membrane caused by prolonged negative pressure (partial vacuum) in the middle ear. Chronic otitis media can lead to permanent conductive hearing loss and, in small children, speech defects because of inability to hear speech sounds properly.

Management:

- Cleaning the ear
- Mopping or suction of the discharge
- Topical antibiotic ear drops for 7-10days
- Oral antibiotics for 7 days
- Treat upper respiratory tract infections, sinusitis

In the absence of fever and severe pain in patients over age 2, analgesics and observation are preferred to antibiotic treatment.

For selected patients, systemic antibiotics (amoxicillin with or without clavulanic acid, erythromycin, trimethoprim-sulfamethoxazole), decongestants, analgesics.

Avoid ototoxic topical antibiotic ear drops (gentamycin, neomycin)

Surgical management:

Myringoplasty:

It is the surgical closure or repair of tympanic membrane perforation

Tympanoplasty:

most common surgical procedure for CSOM. Surgical reconstruction of the tympanic membrane reconstruction of the ossicles.

Ossiculoplasty:

surgical reconstruction of the middle ear bones to restore hearing. Prosthesis made of materials such as Teflon, hydroxyapatite are used to reconnect the ossicles there by re-establishing the sound conduction mechanism.

Myringotomy (surgical puncture of the membrane, with release of pus). In children with recurrent or refractory infections, polyethylene tubes may be placed in the tympanic membrane(s) to aerate the middle ear(s) and allow for escape of purulent secretion.

Cholesteatoma and mastoiditis are treated surgically. Chronic perforation of the tympanic membrane requires surgical repair (tympanoplasty).

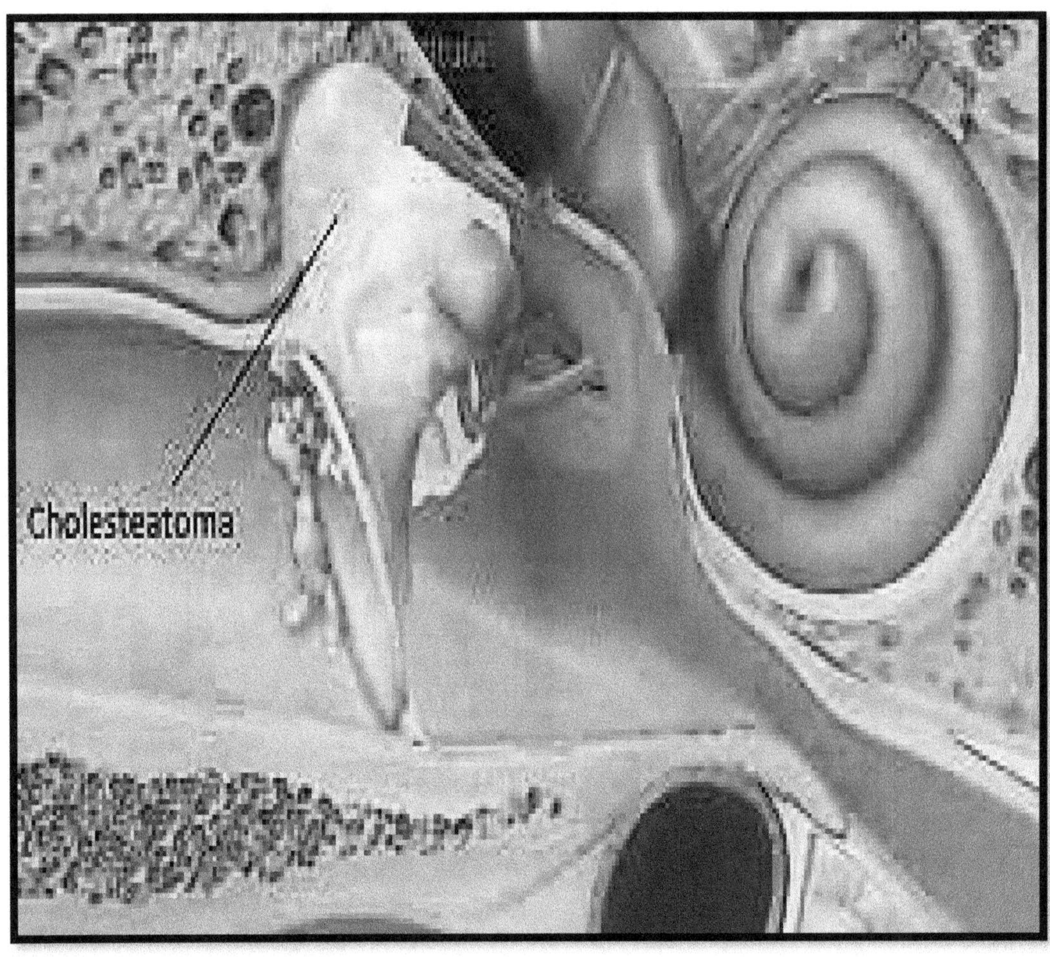

DISORDERS OF THE INNER EAR

Tinnitus

Perception of abnormal sounds in the ear(s) or head.

When pulsatile (simultaneous with heartbeat), it may result from vascular disease (arterial stenosis, aneurysm). Tinnitus is generally a humming or squealing noise heard constantly or intermittently in one or both ears, especially at night when external sounds are at a minimum. It is generally due to degenerative disease of the inner ear, and frequently accompanies sensori neural hearing loss. Common causes are excessive noise exposure and certain medicines. Aspirin and other salicylates at higher doses cause tinnitus lasting only as long as they remain in the body. Other drugs (certain antibiotics) can cause permanent tinnitus. Treatment of tinnitus is generally unsatisfactory but includes masking with other sounds (music, "static" on a radio).

Vertigo

A sense of motion (spinning, falling, floor tipping) when no such motion is occurring.

Causes

 Labyrinthitis, often following respiratory infection and hence often called viral. Degenerative changes in the balance-sensing mechanism of the inner ear. Increased pressure within the endolymphatic sac (Ménière disease). Vascular or neoplastic disease of the inner ear or temporal lobe of the cerebral cortex. Diplopia, head injury, multiple sclerosis, drugs, alcohol.

Signs and symptoms

A feeling of spinning or falling to one side, or a sense that the floor is tipping or rotating, coming on suddenly, often with head movement, and lasting seconds, minutes, hours, days, weeks, or months. When severe, vertigo may make it impossible for the patient to stand or walk, and may be accompanied by nausea and vomiting. There may also be tinnitus and hearing loss.

Physical Examination

 May be essentially normal. The Romberg test (patient standing with eyes closed) may indicate inability to maintain equilibrium. Eyes may show nystagmus.

Treatment:

May be limited to treatment of the underlying cause. In Ménière disease, salt restriction and diuretic therapy may help by reducing the pressure of the endolymph. Medicines such as meclizine and dimenhydrinate may diminish or abolish vertigo temporarily. In some cases of positional vertigo, head manipulation can reduce symptoms by promoting reorientation of the balance mechanism.

MENIERE'S DISEASE

Meniere's disease is a disorder of the inner ear that causes severe dizziness (vertigo), ringing in the ears (tinnitus), hearing loss, and a feeling of fullness or congestion in the ear. Meniere's disease usually affects only one ear.

Attacks of dizziness may come on suddenly or after a short period of tinnitus or muffled hearing. Some people will have single attacks of dizziness separated by long periods of time. Others may experience many attacks closer together over a number of days. Some people with Meniere's disease have vertigo so extreme that they lose their balance and fall. These episodes are called "drop attacks."

Meniere's disease can develop at any age, but it is more likely to happen to adults between 40 and 60 years of age.

Etiological factors

- Exact cause is unknown
- Psychological stress
- Vascular (vasospasm)
- Immunological
- Endocrinological
- Heredity
- Allergy

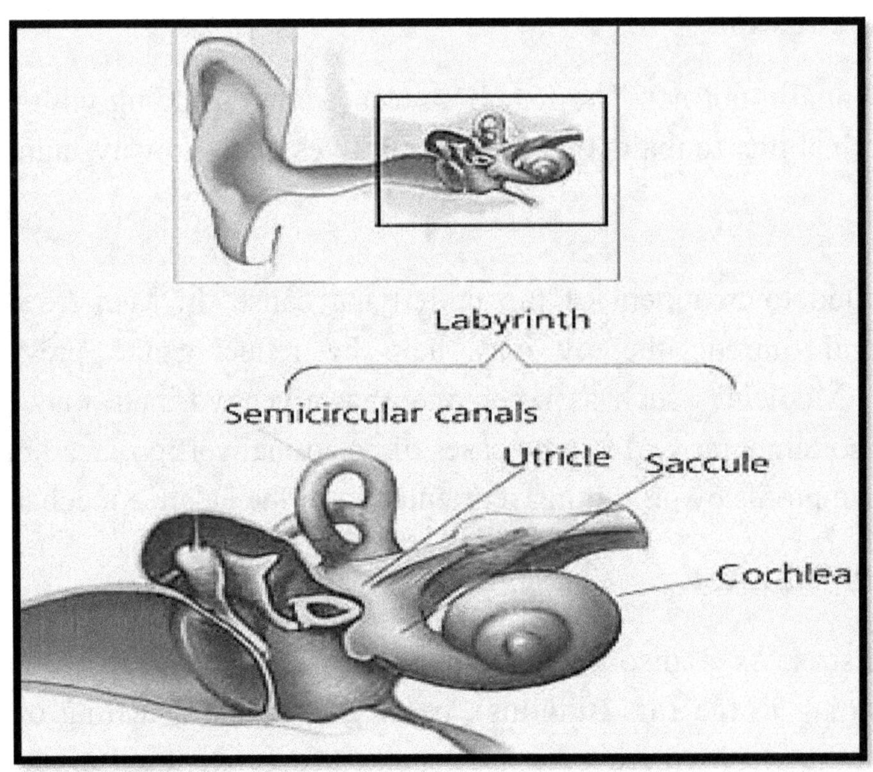

The labyrinth in relation to the ear

The labyrinth is composed of the semicircular canals, the otolithic organs (i.e., utricle and saccule), and the cochlea. Inside their walls (bony labyrinth) are thin, pliable tubes and sacs (membranous labyrinth) filled with endolymph.

The symptoms of Meniere's disease are caused by the buildup of fluid in the compartments of the inner ear, called the labyrinth. The labyrinth contains the organs of balance (the semicircular canals and otolithic organs) and of hearing (the cochlea). It has two sections: the bony labyrinth and the membranous labyrinth. The membranous labyrinth is filled with a fluid called endolymph that, in the balance organs, stimulates receptors as the body moves. The receptors then send signals to the brain about the body's position and movement. In the cochlea, fluid is compressed in response to sound vibrations, which stimulates sensory cells that send signals to the brain.

In Meniere's disease, the endolymph buildup in the labyrinth interferes with the normal balance and hearing signals between the inner ear and the brain. This abnormality causes vertigo and other symptoms of Meniere's disease.

Clinical features

Acute attack

- Unilateral tinnitus
- Vertigo(last for 20 minutes to 2to 3 hours
- Unilateral hearing loss
- nausea, vomiting
- Sensory neural hearing loss
- Nystagmus present during attack and disappear as the vertigo subsides
- Fluctuating hearing loss

Diagnosis

Meniere's disease is most often diagnosed and treated by an otolaryngologist. Diagnosis is based upon your medical history and the presence of:

- Two or more episodes of vertigo lasting at least 20 minutes each

- Tinnitus

- Temporary hearing loss

- A feeling of fullness in the ear

- Caloric test (hypofunction of the labyrinth)

- Audiogram- low frequency sensory neural hearing loss)

- magnetic resonance imaging (MRI) or computed tomography (CT) scans of the brain.

Management

Meniere's disease does not have a cure yet.

- **Medications.** The most disabling symptom of an attack of Meniere's disease is dizziness. Prescription drugs such as meclizine, diazepam, glycopyrolate, and lorazepam can help relieve dizziness and shorten the attack.

- **Salt restriction and diuretics.** Limiting dietary salt and taking diuretics (water pills) help some people control dizziness by reducing the amount of fluid the body retains, which may help lower fluid volume and pressure in the inner ear.

- **Other dietary and behavioral changes.** Some people claim that caffeine, chocolate, and alcohol make their symptoms worse and either avoid or limit them in their diet. Not smoking also may help lessen the symptoms.

- **Cognitive therapy.** Cognitive therapy is a type of talk therapy that helps people focus on how they interpret and react to life experiences. Some people find that cognitive therapy helps them cope better with the unexpected nature of attacks and reduces their anxiety about future attacks.

- **Injections.** Injecting the antibiotic gentamicin into the middle ear helps control vertigo but significantly raises the risk of hearing loss because gentamicin can damage the microscopic hair cells in the inner ear that help us hear. Some doctors inject a corticosteroid instead, which often helps reduce dizziness and has no risk of hearing loss.

- **Pressure pulse treatment.** The U.S. Food and Drug Administration (FDA) recently approved a device for Meniere's disease that fits into the outer ear and delivers intermittent air pressure pulses to the middle ear. The air pressure pulses appear to act on endolymph fluid to prevent dizziness.

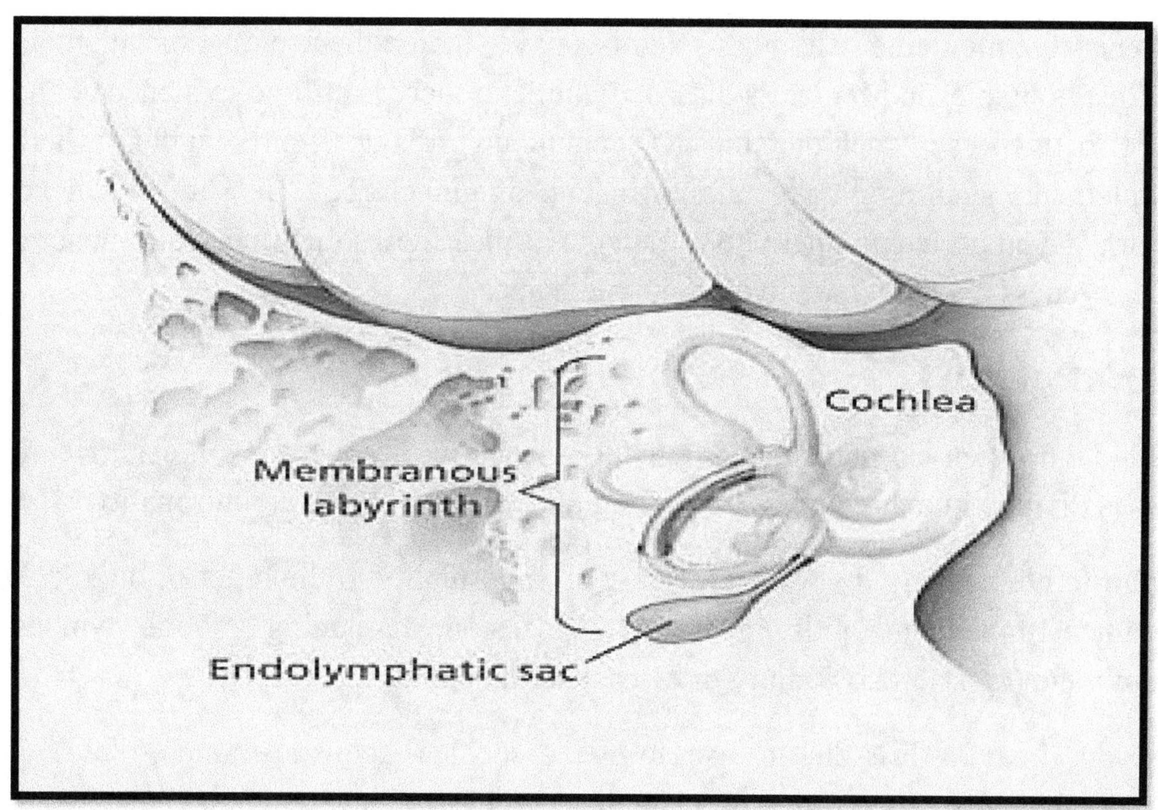

Location of endolymphatic sac

- **Surgery.** Surgery may be recommended when all other treatments have failed to relieve dizziness. Some surgical procedures are performed on the endolymphatic sac to decompress it. Another possible surgery is to cut the vestibular nerve, although this occurs less frequently.

- **Operations designed to influence endolymph production:**

- Sympathectomy from C3 to T3 inclusive of both.

Operations designed to influence endolymph absorption

- Endolymphatic sac decompression and endolymphatic sac CSF shunt

Labyrinthine destruction:

- Labyrinthectomy

- Cryosurgery of labyrinthine

Alternative medicine. Although scientists have studied the use of some alternative medical therapies in Meniere's disease treatment, there is still no evidence to show the effectiveness of such therapies as acupuncture or acupressure, tai chi, or herbal supplements such as gingko biloba, niacin, or ginger root. Be sure to tell your doctor if you are using alternative therapies, since they sometimes can impact the effectiveness or safety of conventional medicines.

HEARING LOSS

Reduction, often permanent, in the acuity of hearing in one or both ears. Hearing loss is divided into three types depending on the location of the abnormality.

Conductive hearing loss due to disease or abnormality in the outer or middle ear: cerumen impaction, otitis media with effusion, hardening of the tympanic membrane (otosclerosis), injury or disease of the ossicles.

Sensory hearing loss due to disease of the cochlea: acoustic trauma, ototoxicity (aminoglycosides, loop diuretics, cisplatin), aging.

Neural hearing loss due to eighth nerve lesions or cerebrovascular disease.

Hearing loss is assessed by audiometry and the Weber and Rinne tests. Treatment is that of the underlying cause, if possible. Generally no treatment is effective.

OTOSCLEROSIS

- Otosclerosis is the slow formation of spongy bone in the otic capsule particularly at the oval window.

- Otoscelrosis is a genetic disease of the otic capsule characterized by deposition of new spongy and vascular bone mainly in the region of stapes fixation and usually conductive hearing loss.

Otosclerosis is a common cause of hearing loss. It is caused by a problem with the tiny bones (ossicles) which transmit vibrations through the middle ear so we can hear sound. Usually both ears are affected in otosclerosis but sometimes only one ear is affected.

Causes:

- 90% bilateral 10% unilateral
- Autosomal dominant trait
- Hereditary
- Racial: most common in Indians While whites, it is rare in negroes

Classification:

- Histological type (common)
- Clinical type
  - Stapedial
  - Cochlear
  - mixed

Symptoms

- Hearing loss(bilateral due to the disruption of the conduction of vibration from the tympanic membrane.

- Speaking softly

- Hearing better in noisy surroundings

- Tinnitus

- Vertigo

- Dizziness and balance problems

Otosclerosis mainly affects the tiny bone (ossicle) called the stirrup (stapes). To have normal hearing, the ossicles need to be able to move freely in response to sound waves. In otosclerosis, abnormal bone material grows around the stapes. The foot of the stapes, where it attaches to the cochlea, is usually where the condition starts. The abnormal bone reduces the movement of the stapes, which reduces the amount of sound that is transferred to the cochlea. The growth of the abnormal bone is very gradual. However, eventually the stapes can become fixed, or fused, with the bone of the cochlea. This can cause severe hearing loss. The hearing loss is known as conductive hearing loss because sound vibrations cannot be conducted (transmitted) from the stapes to the cochlea.

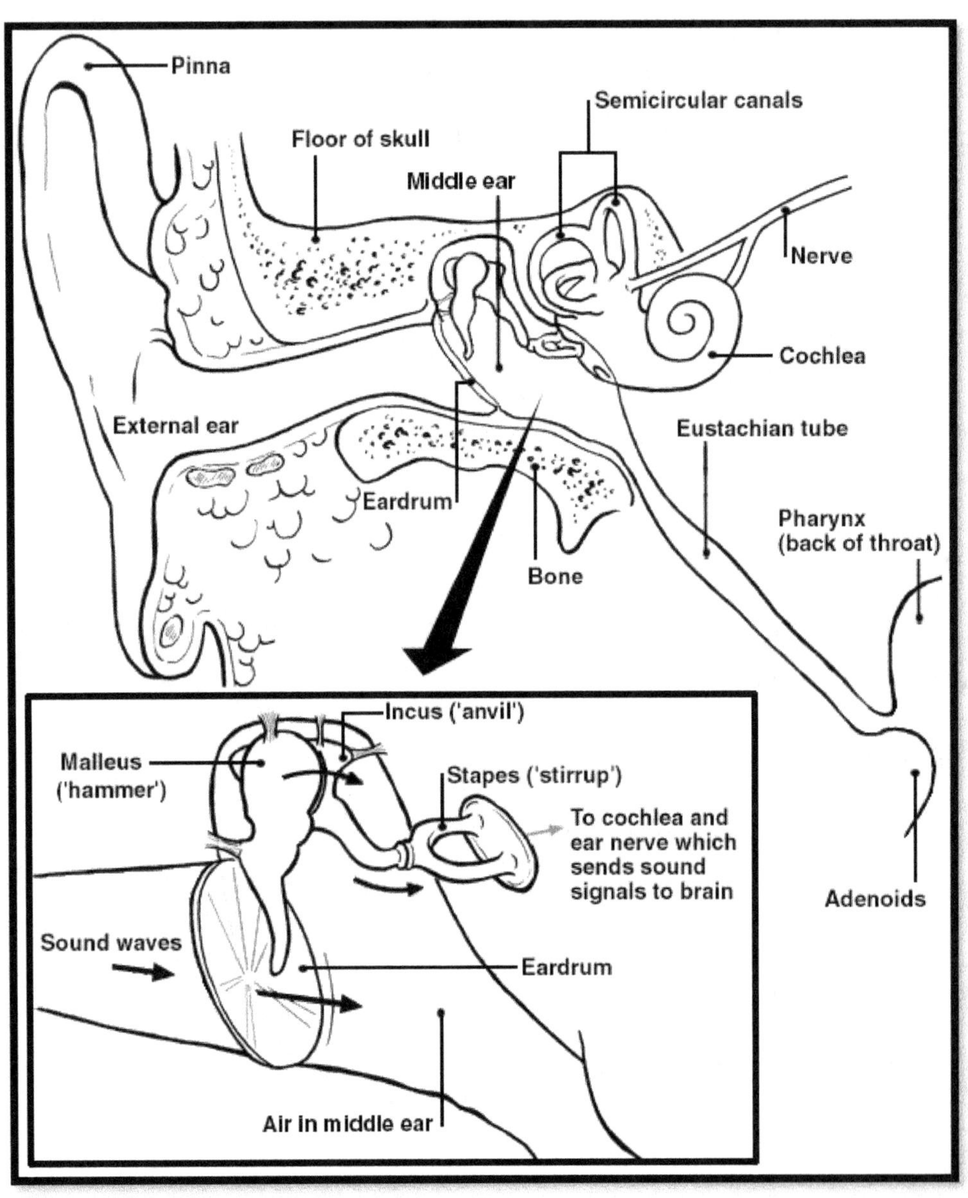

Sound waves come into the outer ear and hit the eardrum.

The sound waves cause the eardrum to vibrate.

The sound vibrations pass from the eardrum to the middle ear bones.

The bones then transmit the vibrations to the cochlea in the inner ear.

The cochlea converts the vibrations to sound signals which are sent along a nerve from the ear to the brain, allowing us to hear.

The semicircular canals in the inner ear contain a fluid that moves around as we move. The movement of the fluid is sensed by tiny hairs in the semicircular canals. These send messages to the brain along the ear (auditory) nerve to the brain to help maintain balance and posture.

Diagnosis

- History collection
- Physical examination
- Rinne test-showing bone conduction lasting longer than air conduction
- Weber test: sound lateralizing to the more affected ear.
- hearing tests which will show a specific pattern of hearing loss in otosclerosis. The specialist may also use a small device that is placed in your ear, called a tympanometer. This can help them look at the movement of the bones within your ear. In otosclerosis, the stirrup (stapes) will move less. This test is very quick and does not cause any pain.
- Audiometry
- Audiogram
- CT scan which will give more information about how severe the otosclerosis is.

HEARING AIDS

when the hearing loss is mild, may not need any treatment. As the disease progresses and hearing loss becomes worse, hearing aids can make a big difference. However, when the hearing loss becomes severe, hearing aids may not be of much help.

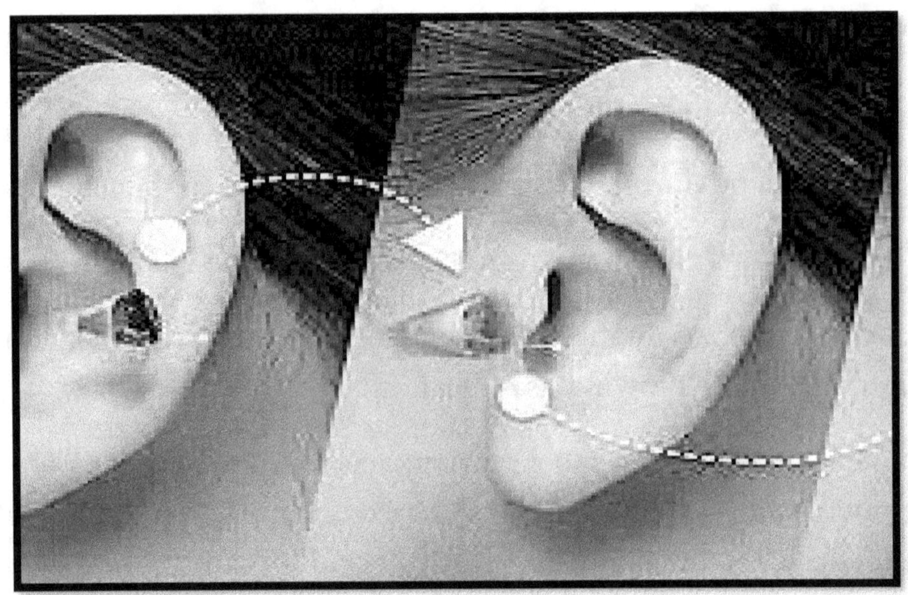

Surgery

Stapedectomy

The most common operation that is done is to replace the stapes with an artificial bone made of plastic or metal. The operation is called a stapedectomy (or sometimes a stapedotomy). In most cases, this operation is successful and restores hearing. It may also reduce the chance of otosclerosis progressing to affect your inner ear.

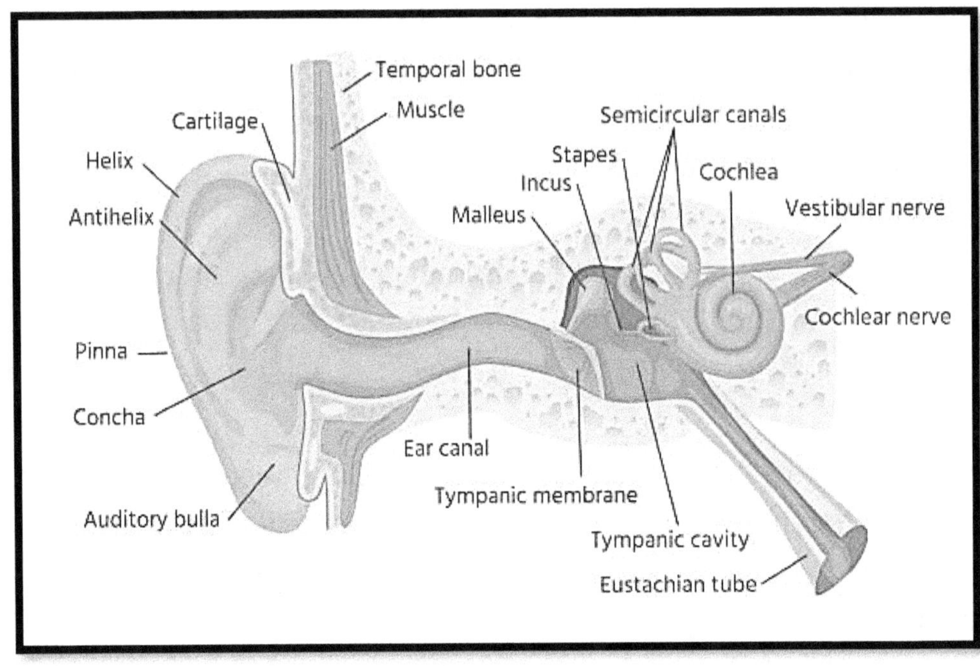

Fluoride tablets

There is some limited evidence that fluoride tablets may possibly slow the progression of the otosclerosis in some cases. They may help to preserve hearing and also help to reduce the symptoms of dizziness and balance problems.

Complications:

- Profound sensorineural hearing loss
- Persistent vertigo

DISEASES OF THE NOSE

CORYZA (COMMON COLD)

Coryza (Common Cold) A common, mild rhinitis caused by viruses.

Causes

Any of numerous viruses, which can be spread readily from person to person. Risk of catching cold may be heightened by exposure to severe winter weather (especially whole-body chilling), drying of indoor air by heating systems, or crowding indoors during the winter.

Signs and symptoms

Headache, nasal stuffiness, runny nose, sneezing, throat irritation, malaise. Occasionally fever, chills, anorexia, and muscle aching.

Physical Examination

Erythema and edema of nasal mucosa. Temperature may be slightly elevated.

Course

Generally self-limited. Sometimes complicated by sinusitis, otitis media, pharyngitis, bronchitis.

Treatment

Purely symptomatic. Oral decongestants are moderately effective. Aspirin, acetaminophen, or ibuprofen relieve discomfort. Rest, fluids. Antihistamines do not decongest, antibiotics.

ALLERGIC RHINITIS (HAY FEVER)

A recurrent, often seasonal, inflammation of the nasal mucous membrane caused by allergy to inhaled materials.

Causes

Sensitivity to pollens, grasses, mold spores, dust mites, animal dander, second-hand cigarette smoke, and other inhalant allergens.

Signs and symptoms

Recurrent or constant nasal congestion and irritation, with copious watery discharge, itching, sneezing (often many times in a row), and itching and watering of the eyes. Symptoms may occur consistently at certain seasons (spring, fall) or, especially when due to house dust, may be perennial.

Physical Examination

Watery, red eyes. Pale or bluish, markedly swollen nasal mucosa. Nasal polyps (massive overgrowths of chronically inflamed mucosa) may be present.

Diagnostic Tests

- Nasal smear shows eosinophils.
- Skin testing or RAST (radio allegro sorbent testing) can identify causative allergens.

Treatment

Decongestants, antihistamines, nasal corticosteroid spray. Avoidance of known allergens when possible. Use of air filters as appropriate. Continued administration of desensitizing antigens often markedly reduces symptoms.

SINUSITIS (RHINOSINUSITIS)

Infection of one or more paranasal sinuses.

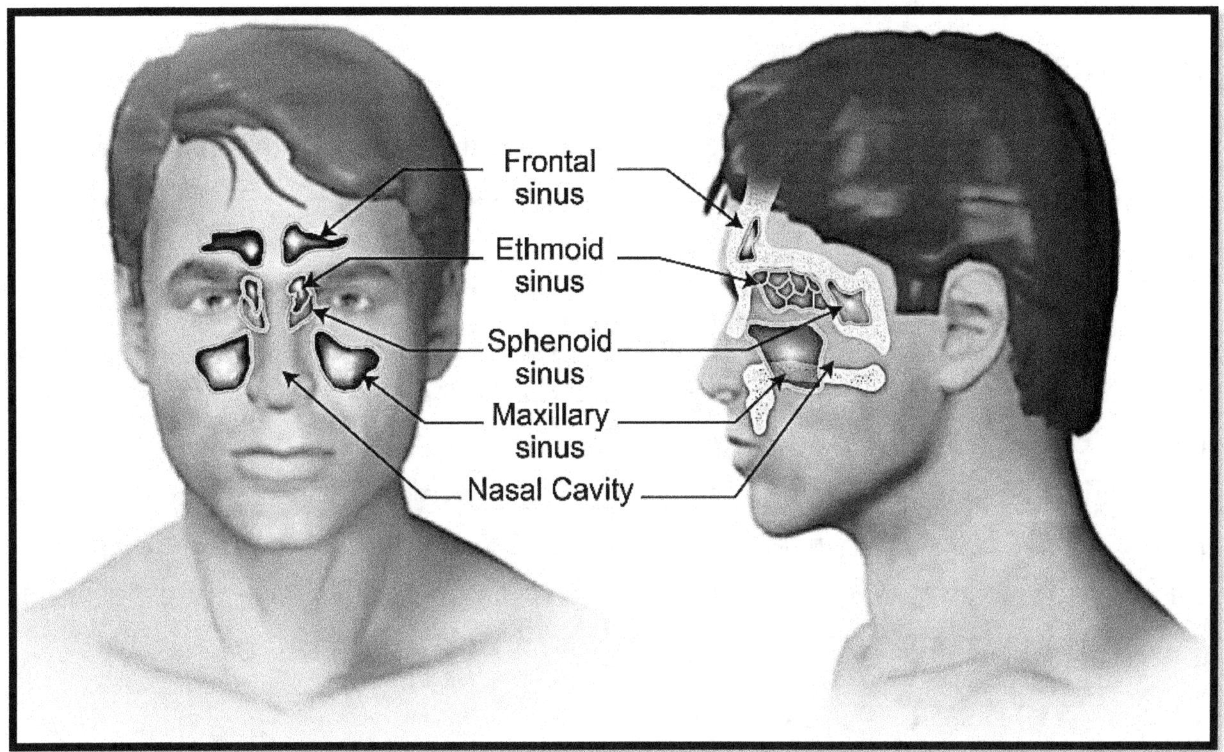

Cause

Involvement of the paranasal sinuses often occurs along with any type of rhinitis, including particularly the common cold. Swelling of the nasal mucosa leads to blockage of the sinus openings, with accumulation of secretions within the sinuses affected. Persons with allergic rhinitis may be subject to recurring episodes of sinusitis due to chronic blockage of sinus openings (ostia). Acute sinusitis is nearly always viral. Recurrent or persistent obstruction to sinus drainage can lead to chronic sinusitis with secondary bacterial infection.

Signs and symptoms

Pressure or pain in one or more sinus cavities, often aggravated by bending forward. Pain may be manifested as a severe headache or may Radiate into the teeth. Purulent or bloody nasal or postnasal discharge may be present. Occasionally fever, chills, and malaise.

Physical Examination

Edema and erythema of nasal mucosa. Purulent discharge in nasal passages or oropharynx (postnasal drip).

Diagnostic Tests

In chronic sinusitis, x-ray or other diagnostic imaging shows thickening of sinus membranes and often presence of fluid within cavities.

Treatment

Decongestant, analgesic. A short course of nasal decongestant spray may help to open and drain sinuses. Control of allergic component if present. When symptoms (severe, persistent pain) or clinical picture (fever, bloody discharge) suggests bacterial infection, an oral antibiotic (amoxicillin, trimethoprim-sulfamethoxazole) is prescribed. Chronic sinusitis may respond to prolonged antibiotic therapy. Surgical procedures can be used to correct anatomic lesions predisposing to sinusitis, or to improve drainage of a chronically infected sinus.

EPISTAXIS (NOSE BLEED)

Bleeding from the nose may be due to nasal trauma, irritation of the mucosa by dust or dry air, upper respiratory infection or allergic rhinitis, or coagulation defect. Treatment of acute nosebleed is by application of direct pressure and, if necessary, topical vasoconstrictor. If bleeding persists or recurs, cautery with silver nitrate or anterior nasal packing may be necessary. Rarely bleeding comes from the posterior nares (usually in middle-aged or elderly patients with hypertension or arteriosclerosis) and requires a posterior nasal pack. Prevention of further nosebleeds may include use of lubricating applications to the mucosa, humidification of air, and avoidance of dusts and other irritants.

ACUTE PHARYNGITIS (SORE THROAT)

Acute inflammation of the throat due to infection.

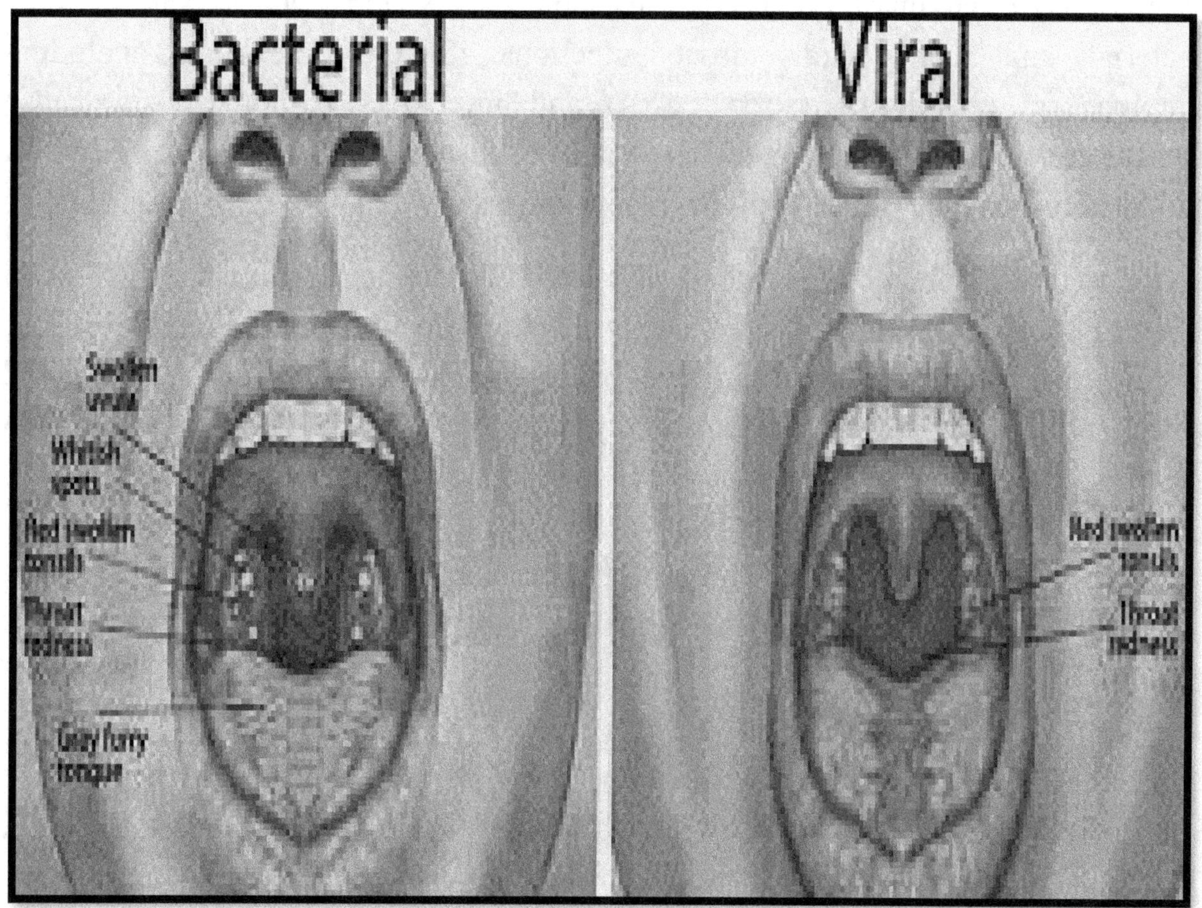

Cause

Usually viruses, including the Epstein Barr virus, which causes infectious mononucleosis. Occasionally bacteria such as Streptococcus pneumonia and Group A beta haemolytic Streptococcus pyogenes ("strep throat"), or fungi such as Candida. Infection with cold viruses may predispose to bacterial infection. Sore throat is more prevalent in cold weather.

Signs and symptoms

Pain, irritation, or a sense of fullness or swelling in the throat, accentuated by swallowing and often radiating to the ears. Fever, painful glandular swelling in the neck.

Physical Examination

May be essentially normal. Fever is often present. Edema and erythema of the oropharynx, often involving the tonsils, soft palate, and uvula, occur in most bacterial and many viral throat infections. Severe infections, including streptococcal pharyngitis (strep throat) and infectious mononucleosis, cause formation of white or grey exudate (consisting of dead tissue, white blood cells, and bacteria) on pharyngeal walls and especially on the tonsils.

A firmly adherent exudate is characteristic of Candida infection (thrush). The presence of vesicles or ulcers suggests viral infection (herpes simplex virus, coxsackievirus). Severe pain and swelling may cause a hollow or "hot potato" voice, and may make swallowing virtually impossible, so that the patient drools to avoid swallowing saliva, and becomes dehydrated from lack of fluid intake. Extreme swelling may compromise the airway. Cervical lymph glands may be swollen and tender. Some strains of beta-hemolytic streptococci cause a widespread red rash (scarlet fever, scarlatina).

Diagnostic Tests

Throat culture or strep screen may identify the causative organism. Blood studies (white blood cell count and differential, anti-streptolysin O titer, heterophile antibodies) help to diagnose strep throat and infectious mononucleosis.

Smears or scrapings of exudate can confirm presence of Candida.

Course

Viral sore throat runs its course within a week or two. Occasionally it becomes complicated by streptococcal infection, which may lead to acute rheumatic fever. It may also progress to otitis media, acute or chronic tonsillitis, or lower respiratory infection. Peri tonsillar abscess **(quinsy)** is a severe bacterial infection developing above and behind one tonsil and causing extreme pain and swelling, with deviation of the uvula away from the affected side.

Treatment

Acute viral pharyngitis requires no treatment except analgesics, gargles, soothing lozenges, and perhaps a soft diet. Adrenal corticosteroid may be administered orally or by injection for severe pain and swelling. If streptococcal infection is diagnosed, a 10-day course of an antibiotic known to be able to eradicate streptococci (such as penicillin V, erythromycin, or cephalexin) is mandatory.

Candidal oropharyngitis (thrush) is treated with topical or systemic antifungal medicine. The treatment of peritonsillar abscess is surgical drainage.

OBSTRUCTIVE SLEEP APNEA (OSA)

A disorder in which breathing is repeatedly interrupted during sleep by intermittent obstruction of the airway.

Cause

Lax, excessively bulky, or malformed pharyngeal tissues (soft palate, uvula, and sometimes tonsils). Obesity, hypothyroidism, cigarette smoking, alcohol, and some medicines (particularly benzodiazepines) are predisposing factors. The swallowing reflex may be impaired during sleep. The condition is twice as common in men. Incidence increases with advancing age.

Signs and symptoms

Loud snoring and recurrent episodes of apnea (respiratory arrest) during sleep followed by gasping inspiration with partial or complete arousal. The period of apnea may last for 10-120 seconds, and may be accompanied by sinus bradycardia or atrioventricular block.

Physical Examination

The shape and caliber of upper respiratory passages may be abnormal.

Diagnostic Tests

Polysomnography (continuous monitoring of heart rate, respiratory action and air flow, eye movements, and electroencephalogram during sleep), supplemented by recording of chin movements and arterial oxygen saturation.

Course

Nocturnal hypoxemia (deficiency of oxygen in blood) and shallow, non-refreshing sleep may lead to daytime lethargy, difficulties with memory and concentration, and even personality change and accident-proneness. About 15% of persons with OSA develop sustained pulmonary hypertension.

Treatment

Weight loss, smoking cessation, avoidance of alcohol and benzodiazepines. An appliance worn inside the mouth may reduce symptoms by holding the lower jaw in a forward position. The nightly use of continuous positive airway pressure (CPAP), which provides a steady flow of room air at low pressure through the nose to overcome intermittent upper respiratory obstruction, is often effective.

Surgical trimming and reshaping of the uvula and soft palate can be performed by laser or radiofrequency ablation under local anesthesia.

A more elaborate procedure is mandibular osteotomy with genio glossus muscle advancement.

CHAPTER - 4

NURSING MANAGEMENT OF ENT DISORDERS

When caring for a patient with an ENT disorder, you're likely to use several nursing diagnoses repeatedly. These commonly used diagnoses appear here, along with appropriate nursing interventions and rationales.

Impaired swallowing

Related to pain and inflammation, Impaired swallowing may be associated with such conditions as pharyngitis, tonsillitis, and laryngitis.

Expected outcomes

Patient can swallow.

Patient maintains adequate hydration.

Patient exhibits effective airway clearance.

Nursing interventions and rationales

- Elevate the head of the bed 90 degrees after food or fluid intake and at least 45 degrees at all other times to promote swallowing and prevent aspiration.
- Position the patient on his side while recumbent to decrease the risk of aspiration. Have suction equipment available in case aspiration occurs.
- Assess swallowing function frequently, especially before meals, to prevent aspiration.
- Administer pain medication before meals to enhance swallowing ability.
- Provide a liquid to soft diet, and consult with the dietitian as necessary to promote less painful swallowing.
- Provide mouth care frequently to remove secretions and enhance comfort and appetite.
- If the patient can't swallow fluids, notify the practitioner and administer I.V. fluids as ordered to maintain hydration.

Disturbed sensory perception (auditory)

Related to altered auditory reception or transmission, Disturbed sensory perception (auditory) may be associated with such conditions as otitis media, mastoiditis, otosclerosis, Meniere's disease, and labyrinthitis.

Expected outcomes

- Patient understands that progressive hearing loss is caused by the disease.
- Patient can communicate.

Nursing interventions and rationales

- Assess the patient's degree of hearing impairment, and determine the best way to communicate with him (for example, using gestures, lip reading, or written words) to ensure adequate patient care.
- When talking to a hearing-impaired person, speak clearly and slowly in a normal to deep voice and offer concise explanations of procedures to include the patient in his own care.
- Provide sensory stimulation by using tactile and visual stimuli to help compensate for hearing loss.
- Encourage the patient to express feelings of concern and loss for his hearing deficit, and be available to answer questions. This helps him accept his loss, clears up misconceptions, and reduces anxiety.
- Encourage the patient to use his hearing aid as directed to enhance auditory function.
- Upon discharge, teach him to watch for visual cues in the environment, such as traffic lights and flashing lights on emergency vehicles, to avoid injury.

Ineffective airway clearance

Related to nasopharyngeal obstruction, Ineffective airway clearance may be associated with such conditions as nasal papillomas, adenoid hyperplasia, nasal polyps, pharyngitis, and tonsillitis.

Expected outcomes

- Patient has clear nasal airways.
- Patient sleeps with normal oxygen saturation.

- Patient is free from infection.
- Patient is free from complications.

Nursing interventions and rationales

- Assess respiratory status (including rate, depth, and stridor) at least every 4 hours to detect early signs of compromise.
- Position the patient with the head of his bed elevated 45 to 90 degrees to promote drainage of secretions and aid breathing and chest expansion.
- Suction upper airways as needed to help remove secretions.
- Have emergency equipment at the bedside in case of airway obstruction.
- Encourage the patient to cough and deep-breathe every 2 hours to help loosen secretions in his lungs.
- Encourage the patient to drink at least 3 qt (3 L) of fluid per day to ensure adequate hydration and loosen secretions.

Common ENT disorders

Hearing loss, laryngitis, otitis externa, otitis media, and sinusitis are common ENT disorders.

Hearing loss

Impaired hearing, the most common disability in the United States, results from a mechanical or nervous system impediment to the transmission of sound waves. Hearing loss is further defined as an inability to perceive the range of sounds audible to an individual with normal hearing. Types of hearing loss include congenital hearing loss, sudden deafness, noise-induced hearing loss, and presbycusis (age-related hearing loss.

The major forms of hearing loss are classified as:

conductive, in which transmission of sound impulses from the external ear to the junction of the stapes and oval window is interrupted

sensorineural, in which impaired cochlear or acoustic (CN VIII) nerve function prevents transmission of sound impulses within the inner ear or brain

mixed, in which conductive and sensorineural transmission dysfunction combine.

Although congenital hearing loss may produce no obvious signs of hearing impairment at birth, deficient response to auditory stimuli usually becomes apparent within 2 to 3 days. As the child grows older, hearing loss impairs speech development.

Ear, nose, and throat disorders: Loud and long

Noise-induced hearing loss causes sensorineural damage, the extent of which depends on the duration and intensity of the noise. Initially, the patient loses perception of certain frequencies (around 4,000 Hz) but, with continued exposure, he eventually loses perception of all frequencies.

Presbycusis usually produces tinnitus, with progressive decline in overall hearing and the ability to understand the spoken word.

Patient, family, and occupational histories and a complete audiologic examination usually provide ample evidence of hearing loss and suggest possible causes or predisposing factors.

Weber and Rinne tests as well as specialized audiologic tests differentiate between conductive and sensorineural hearing loss.

Auditory evoked reponses, imaging studies, and electronystagmography help to evaluate disorders, such as vertigo, neuromas, and tinnitus.

To treat sudden deafness, the underlying cause must be promptly identified. Educating patients and health care professionals about the many causes of sudden deafness can greatly reduce the incidence of this problem.

Ear, nose, and throat disorders: Deafness and decibels

For individuals whose hearing loss was induced by noise levels greater than 90 dB for several hours, treatment includes: overnight rest, which usually restores normal hearing unless the patient was repeatedly exposed to such noise speech and hearing rehabilitation as the patient's hearing deteriorates, because hearing aids are rarely helpful.

Nurses role

- When talking to a patient with hearing loss who can read lips, stand directly in front of him, with the light on your face, and speak slowly and distinctly.
- Assess the degree of hearing impairment without shouting.
- Approach the patient within his visual range, and get his attention by raising your arm or waving; touching him may unnecessarily startle him.
- Write instructions on a tablet, if necessary, to make sure the patient understands.
- If the patient is learning to use a hearing aid, provide emotional support and encouragement.
- Inform other staff members and hospital personnel of the patient's disability and his established method of communication.
- Ear, nose, and throat disorders: Seeing clues
- Make sure the patient is in an area where he can observe unit activities and persons approaching, because a patient with hearing loss depends on visual clues.
- Evaluate the patient. Make sure he expresses that his hearing loss has resolved or stabilized, is able to maintain communication with others, and exhibits decreased anxiety.
- Make sure the patient and his family understand the importance of wearing protective devices while in a noisy environment. (See Hearing loss teaching tips.)
- To prevent noise-induced hearing loss, the public must be educated about the dangers of noise exposure and come to insist on the use, as mandated by law, of protective devices, such as earplugs, during occupational exposure to noise.
- To help prevent congenital hearing loss, pregnant women need to understand the dangers of exposure to drugs, chemicals, and infection — especially rubella — during pregnancy.

Hearing loss teaching tips

- Explain the cause of hearing loss and the medical or surgical treatment options.
- Teach the patient who just received a hearing aid how it works and how to maintain it.
- Emphasize the danger of excessive exposure to noise, and encourage the use of protective devices in a noisy environment.

LARYNGITIS

Laryngitis is an inflammation of the vocal cords. Acute laryngitis may occur as an isolated infection or as part of a generalized bacterial or viral upper respiratory tract infection. Repeated attacks of acute laryngitis cause inflammatory changes associated with chronic laryngitis.

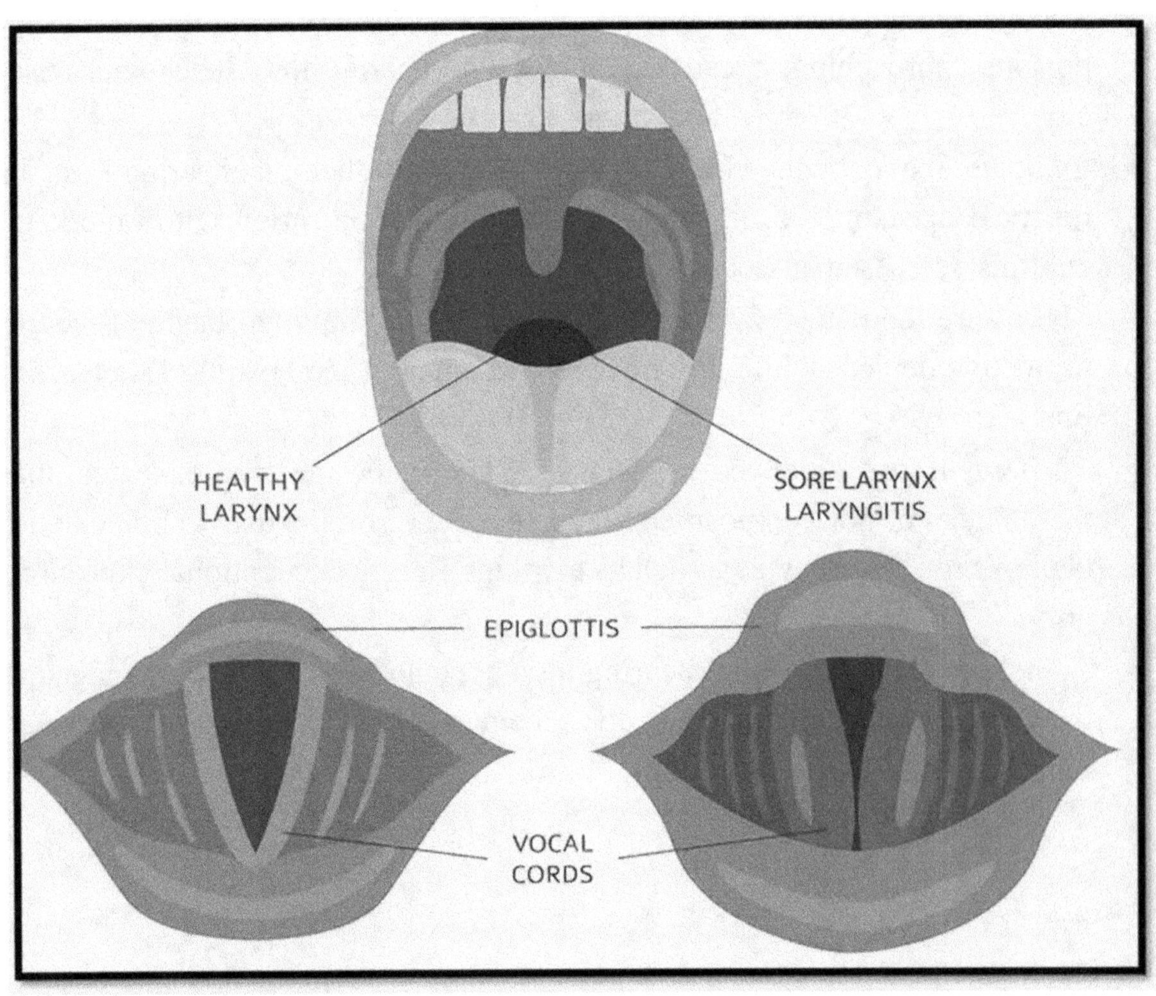

causes

Acute laryngitis results from infection, excessive use of the voice, inhalation of smoke or fumes, or aspiration of caustic chemicals. Chronic laryngitis results from upper respiratory tract disorders (such as sinusitis, bronchitis, nasal polyps, or allergy), mouth breathing, smoking, gastroesophageal reflux, constant exposure to dust or other irritants, alcohol abuse, or cancer of the larynx.

Edema of the vocal cords caused by irritation (from an infection, lesion, or overuse of the voice or other cause) impairs the normal mobility of the vocal cords, causing an abnormal sound.

look for Signs and symptoms of laryngitis include:

- hoarseness (persistent hoarseness in chronic laryngitis)
- changes in the character of the voice
- pain (especially when swallowing or speaking)
- a dry cough, fever, malaise, dyspnea, throat clearing, restlessness, or laryngeal edema.

Indirect laryngoscopy confirms the diagnosis by revealing exudate and red, inflamed, and occasionally hemorrhagic vocal cords, with rounded (not sharp) edges. Bilateral swelling that restricts movement but doesn't cause paralysis also may be apparent. Video stroboscopy shows the movement of the vocal cords.

Treatment of laryngitis includes

- resting the voice (primary treatment)
- symptomatic care, such as an analgesic and throat lozenges (for viral infection)
- antibiotic therapy (bacterial infection), usually with cefuroxime (Ceftin)
- identification and elimination of underlying cause (chronic laryngitis)
- possible hospitalization (in severe acute laryngitis)
- possible tracheotomy if laryngeal edema results in airway obstruction
- drug therapy, which may include antacids, histamine-2 blockers, antibiotics, and systemic steroids.

Nurses role

- Tell the patient to refrain from talking to avoid straining the vocal cords and allow vocal cord inflammation to decrease.
- If the patient is hospitalized, place a sign over his bed to remind others of talking restrictions and mark the intercom panel so other hospital personnel are aware that the patient can't answer.
- Provide a pad and pencil or a slate for communication.
- Provide an ice collar, a throat irrigant, and cold fluids for comfort.
- Evaluate the patient. Make sure he isn't hoarse or in pain; doesn't have a fever; doesn't need a tracheotomy; understands the need to stop smoking, maintain humidification, and complete his antibiotic therapy; and modifies his environment appropriately to prevent recurrence.

Laryngitis teaching tips

- Suggest that the patient maintain adequate humidification by using a vaporizer or humidifier during the winter, avoiding air conditioning during the summer (because it dehumidifies), using medicated throat lozenges, and avoiding smoking and smoky environments.
- Teach the patient about prescribed medication, including dosage, frequency, and adverse effects.
- Instruct the patient to complete prescribed antibiotic therapy.
- If the patient has chronic laryngitis, obtain a detailed patient history to help determine the cause.
- Encourage modification of habits that can cause the disorder.
- Advise the patient to avoid crowds and people with upper respiratory tract infections.

CHAPTER - 5

REHABILITATION AND FOLLOW UP FOR ENT DISORDERS

Aural rehabilitation is defined holistically as the reduction of hearing-loss-induced deficits of function, activity, participation, and quality of life through a combination of sensory management, instruction, perceptual training, and counselling.

GOALS

This goal can be addressed through a combination of:

- sensory management to optimize auditory function,
- instruction in the use of technology and control of the listening environment,
- perceptual training to improve speech perception and communication, and
- counseling to enhance participation, and deal both emotionally and practically with residual limitations.

Training programs must provide budding audiologists with knowledge and skills in this area, including:

- an understanding of, and sensitivity to, the psychosocial issues surrounding acquired hearing loss; appropriate interactive styles;
- the ability to recognize when there is a need for services beyond their expertise and/or scope of practice;
- the realization that they do not treat hearing loss in people–they serve people with hearing loss

The cochlear implant

The cochlear implant is a medical device designed to enable a person with a severe-to-profound sensorineural hearing loss to detect speech and environmental sounds. The internal portion of the device is surgically placed under the skin behind the ear with an electrode array inserted into the hearing organ (the cochlea). The device bypasses the damaged hearing organ and stimulates usable nerve fibers that go to the brain. Through this stimulation, people can often learn to listen and understand speech and environmental sounds. The external portion of the device includes a sound processor, cord, transmitter, and microphone and is worn like a behind-the-ear hearing aid.

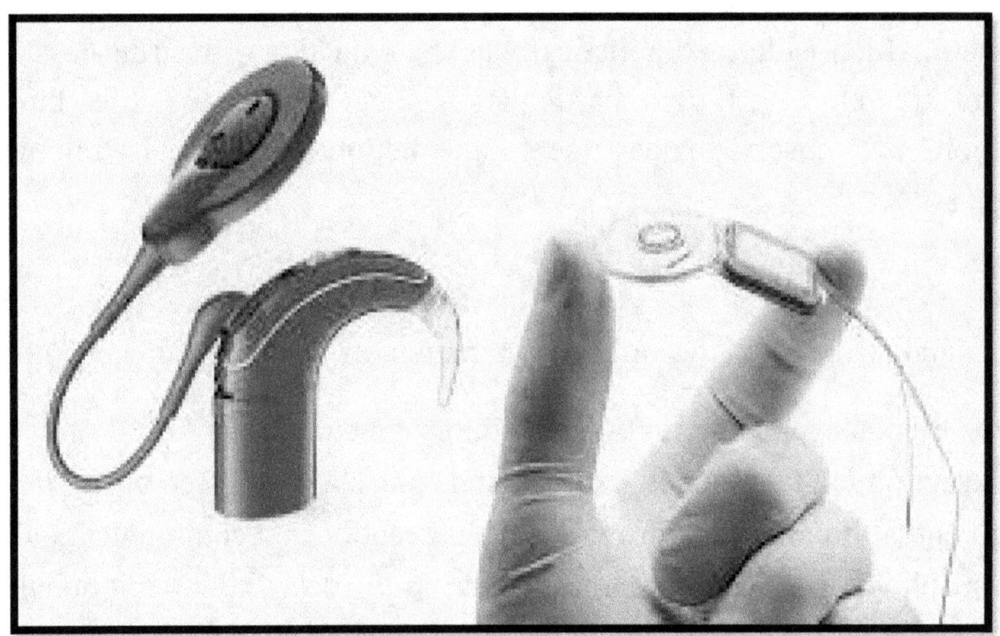

Benefits of the Cochlear Implant

Cochlear implant recipients may feel more connected to the world around them. They can hear environmental sounds like birds singing, telephones ringing, and cars approaching. They can also learn to detect and understand speech. This connection to their environment often results in feeling less isolated and more independent and self-confident.

Children who generally benefit the most from cochlear implants are those who are deaf for a short period of time, in good auditory training programs, and have families who are strongly committed to the training process. Children continue to experience hearing improvement for years after the implant is inserted.

As for adults who have already developed spoken language, the cochlear implant provides an opportunity to regain personal communication. It enables the ability to have a sense of security, more freedom, and an opportunity to be more socially engaged. While there is no definitive test to predetermine the extent of results, nearly all patients show significant hearing improvement.

Candidacy Criteria

Candidacy determination can be a complex process. The guidelines below serve as a broad indication for cochlear implantation and not as the only cases for which a cochlear implant would be appropriate.

- Children 12 months of age and older with limited or no progress in auditory development
- Adults 18 years of age and older with limited or no benefit from hearing aids
- Individuals with severe to profound sensorineural hearing loss in one or both ears
- Individuals in good general health
- Individuals willing and motivated to be actively involved in therapy
- If you are interested in learning more about cochlear implant candidacy requirements, please contact us. We will provide additional information, ask you to complete a cochlear implant survey, and discuss treatment options with you.

Candidacy Evaluation Process

Adults

• Audiological evaluation (hearing assessment)

• CT scans or MRI (specialized x-ray to evaluate the hearing anatomy)

• Medical evaluation (determines if the patient has conditions that would prohibit surgery)

Children

• Sedated auditory brainstem response and otoacoustic emissions tests (objective measures of hearing sensitivity)

• Speech-language evaluation (assessment of communication abilities with hearing aids and discussion of communication goals)

• Cognitive and psychological evaluation (understanding expectations and coping strategies for the patient and family)

• Developmental evaluation (assessment of developmental milestones and capacity to learn)

• Educational assessment (child's school is contacted regarding educational placement, support, and training on cochlear implants)

Hearing for the First Time with an Implant

During the first six months, the patient returns frequently for reprogramming to help the ear adjust to the new stimulation. Usually after the first six months, the patient will return every six months for the first three years to fine tune and update the sound processor's software. After three years, patients return on an annual basis.

Importance of Therapy

For both children and adults who have been without sound, therapy is critical for successful use and understanding of speech.

Adults may have a lifetime of auditory memories to draw upon and usually learn to recognize the new speech sounds in a relatively short period of time. Therapy consists of listening to individual speech sounds, words, phrases, sentences, and conversations; practice to improve communication situations and counselling.

Children often have little or no listening experiences. Without intensive speech therapy and education, these children will not benefit from the cochlear implant. According to the National Institute of Health (NIH), "access to optimal educational and rehabilitation services is important to adults and is critical to children to maximize the benefits available from cochlear implantation."

Vestibular and balance disorders

Patients suffering from vestibular disorders often experience problems with vertigo, dizziness and visual disturbance and/or imbalance. Secondary problems can also arise, such as nausea, vomiting, inability to concentrate, fatigue, anxiety and depression. These symptoms can be disruptive to everyday life. Activities that were simple before the vestibular disorder may become difficult. Patients often develop a more sedentary lifestyle to avoid worsening symptoms. A sedentary lifestyle can contribute to weakness, joint stiffness and a decrease in physical health and endurance to perform daily activities.

Treatment may include medication, in-clinic procedures, surgery along with Vestibular Rehabilitation Therapy (VRT), an exercise-based program to reduce symptoms related to inner ear and balance disorders.

Dizziness can be a description of multiple types of symptoms. The physician usually tries to categorize dizziness into one of the four categories below:

Vertigo: temporary, episodic or persistent sensation of spinning dizziness, sometimes accompanied by sweating, nausea, vomiting, headaches, hearing loss, tinnitus (ringing in the ear), sound sensitivity or light sensitivity; symptoms can come and go, and each episode may last from minutes to hours

Light headedness: sensation of impending loss of consciousness, sometimes accompanied by sensory disturbances, orthostatic hypotension, cardiac arrhythmia and panic attacks

Disequilibrium: imbalance or unsteadiness caused by diminished vision, loss of vestibular function, defects in proprioception and motor dysfunction

Oscillopsia: illusion of visual motion when the eyes are open

Skull base lesions

Skull base lesions vary in size, location, and severity, so every case is unique.

Acoustic Neuroma

Acoustic neuroma (vestibular schwannoma) is a non-cancerous tumor that may develop from an overproduction of Schwann cells that press on hearing and balance nerves in the inner ear. Schwann cells are cells that normally wrap around and support nerve fibers. If the tumor becomes large, it can press on the facial nerve or brain structure. Unilateral acoustic neuromas affect only one ear and occur most often between the ages of 30 and 60. Bilateral acoustic neuromas affect both ears and are hereditary, caused by a genetic disorder called neurofibromatosis-2.

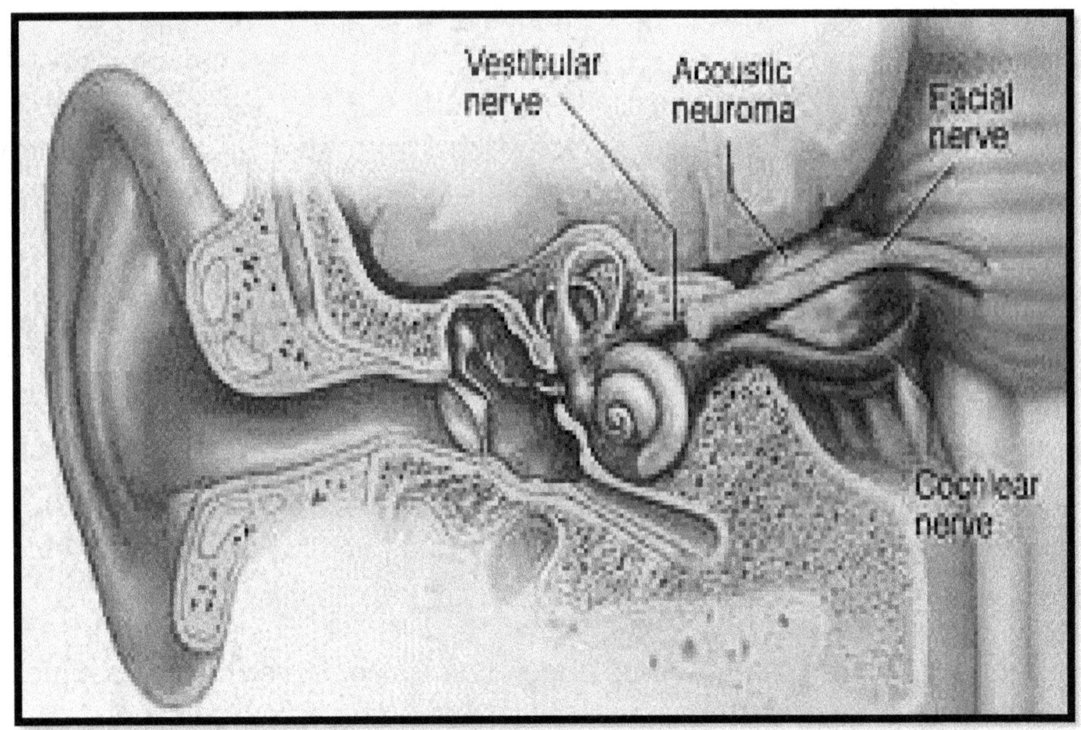

Symptoms may include hearing loss, feeling of fullness in the ear, tinnitus (ringing), dizziness, balance problems, facial numbness and tingling, facial nerve paralysis, headaches, and mental confusion. In rare cases it can be life threatening and require immediate medical treatment.

Because symptoms of acoustic neuromas resemble other middle- and inner-ear conditions, they may be difficult to diagnose. Preliminary diagnostic procedures include an ear exam and a hearing test. A magnetic resonance imaging (MRI) scan may help to determine the tumor's location and size. Early diagnosis offers the best opportunity for successful treatment. Treatment is determined based on age, overall health, medical history, tumor size, hearing ability, and expectations for disease progression. Treatment may include observation with serial imaging, microsurgery, or stereotactic radiation (Gamma Knife).

MENINGIOMA

Meningioma is a tumor that grows in the meninges (layers of tissue that cover the brain and spinal cord). They are usually benign so, unlike cancerous tumors, they don't tend to spread to distant parts of the body. Meningioma tumors occur more often than cancerous brain tumors. They are often discussed alongside brain tumors and can cause neurological problems. As these tumors grow, they can compress the brain and spinal cord, leading to serious complications. Children rarely get meningiomas tumors, and they are more common in older adults. Women are more likely to get them than men.

Symptoms may not develop until the tumor has become large. Symptoms vary based on the tumor's location and can include vision or hearing loss, seizures, trouble thinking clearly, trouble walking, loss of smell, weakness in an arm or leg, headaches, or nausea.

Meningioma is diagnosed with an MRI, CT scan, or biopsy. Stereotactic radiation or microsurgical removal is recommended when symptoms are severe, or the tumor is growing. In some cases, like if the tumor is too close to a vital brain structure or blood vessel, surgical removal may be too risky. Meningioma may grow back after surgery, so radiation therapy may be recommended to help prevent another meningioma from developing.

Treatment for Tinnitus

Treatment is determined based on age, overall health, medical history, extent of the disease, and expectations for progression.

Treatments to address symptoms include:

- Hearing aids
- Cochlear implants
- Maskers (small electronic device to make ringing seem softer)
- Medication
- Counseling
- Relaxation
- Surgery (for tumors, abnormal blood flow, or ear muscle spasms)

AFTER EAR SURGERY INSTRUCTIONS

Reasons to Call Immediately

- Temperature greater than 101.5 F
- Difficulty eating or drinking

- Difficulty breathing
- Chest pain
- Severe headache with neck stiffness
- Persistent nausea and vomiting
- Oozing, milky, thick, green or foul-smelling drainage
- Worsening redness, swelling, pain
- Worsening dizziness
- Head dressing saturated with blood
- Incision does not stop bleeding
- Any other questions or concern

Wound Care

- For one to two days, there may be a small amount of blood oozing from the incision inside the ear canal and/or behind the ear. doctor will indicate when the head dressing and gauze can be removed
- For one to two weeks, some blood (or brown, pink, yellow, black or clear fluid) may drain from your ear canal; cotton in the ear can be changed as needed if it is soaked with drainage; stop using cotton if there is no drainage
- Ear packing may fall out, but do not remove it; apply ear drops directly to packing
- In one week, skin tape covering the incision may be removed if it has not fallen off
- Do not remove any stitches, as they dissolve on their own

Common Symptoms

- Pain around the surgical site (improves with time but may last up to two weeks)
- Numbness around the incision and ear (gradually improves with time)
- Clicking, popping, pulsing, ringing, or other sounds
- Soreness or bruising of the lips, eyelids, and shoulders
- Jaw, neck or throat pain
- Headaches and fatigue

Medications

- Resume home medication, unless instructed otherwise
- Follow prescription instructions for application procedure, frequency, and quantity of ear drops
- Acetaminophen (Tylenol) or ibuprofen (Motrin) as needed for pain
- Prescription narcotics (Norco, Percocet) for breakthrough pain only (some narcotics have acetaminophen included, so do not take acetaminophen at the same time)
- Call the clinic if you need narcotic pain medications
- Fiber and stool softeners (docusate) may help with constipation from pain medications
- Anti-nausea medications may be prescribed for dizziness with nausea and/or vomiting

Showering

- ALWAYS keep the inside of the ear dry
- Shower or bathe 48 hours after surgery, but do not soak or scrub the wound
- Place a cotton ball coated with Vaseline or an earplug in the outside bowl of the ear (don't use cotton without lubricant or push on packing inside the ear)
- If water gets in, dab with a dry towel; don't place anything inside the ear canal
- Dry incisions immediately after showering and apply moisturizing lotion (Aquaphor, Cetaphil) or antibiotic ointment (if prescribed) over incisions until they are fully healed; no need to apply lotion when incision is covered by tape, but apply when the tape falls off

Activity Restrictions

- doctor will indicate when it's okay to return to work or fly
- To decrease chance of bleeding, don't lift more than 20 pounds or strain for two weeks
- Do not strain on the toilet or blow your nose (sneeze with your mouth open)
- Take care when driving, walking, and showering, as there may be dizziness or imbalance for days to weeks after surgery

Diet

Consume healthy food and maintain hydration by drinking plenty of water. Food may taste different or there may be decreased taste for weeks to months.

Ear Irrigation

Ear irrigation is the process of flushing the external ear canal with sterile water or sterile saline. It is used to treat patients who complain of foreign body or cerumen (ear wax) impaction.

Purpose:

- The purpose of ear irrigation is to remove earwax that is obstructing the ear canal or to remove a foreign object lodged in the ear canal.
- Ear irrigation is most commonly performed on those who experience a wax buildup that has impaired **hearing** and irritated the outer ear canal.

Objective

- To cleanse the canal of discharge, to soften and remove impacted cerumen, or to dislodge a foreign object.

Indication

- Cerumen impaction or a foreign body in the ear.

Contraindication

- This procedure is contraindicated when the auditory canal is obstructed by a vegetable foreign body such as pea, bean, or corn kernel. These vegetable absorb moisture, causing them to swell. The procedure is also contraindicated if the patient has a cold, fever, ear infection or unknown injury or rupture of the tympanic membrane.

Nursing alert: Avoid dropping or squiring on the ear drum. Never use more than 500 ml of solution. If the tympanic membrane is ruptured, check with the doctor before irrigating. Monitor temperature of solution carefully. Forceful instillation of the solution can rupture the tympanic membrane. If pain or dizziness occurs, stop the procedure.

Charting

- Document the date and type of irrigation and which ear was irrigated. Also note volume and type of solution and the appearance of the return flow

After care

- Discard equipment in appropriate area.

- Wash your hands.

Equipments

- Prescribed irrigating solution warmed to 37 C (98.6 F), irrigation set (container and irrigating or bulb syringe), emesis basin, cotton-tipped applicator, cotton balls, waterproof pad.

Nursing Interventions & Rationale

Nursing Interventions	Rationale
Explain the procedure to the client.	Explanation facilitates cooperation and provides reassurance for the patient.
Assemble the equipment. Protect the client and bed linens with a moisture proof pad.	This provides for an organized approach to the task.
Wash your hands.	Handwashing deters the spread of microorganisms.
Have the client sit up or lie with the	Gravity causes the irrigating solution

head tilted toward the side of the affected ear. Have the client support a basin under the ear to receive the irrigating solution.	to flow from the ear to the basin.
Clean the pinna and the meatus at the auditory canal as necessary with the normal saline or the irrigating solution.	Materials lodged on the pinna and the meatus may be washed into the ear.
Fill the bulb syringe with solution. If an irrigating container is used, allow air to escape from the tubing.	Air forced into the ear canal is noisy and therefore unpleasant for the client.
Straightening the auditory canal by pulling the pinna down and back for an infant and up and back for an adult	Straightening the ear canal aids in allowing solution to reach all areas of the ears easily.
Direct a steady, slow stream of solution against the roof of the auditory canal, using only sufficient force to remove secretions. Do not occlude the auditory canal with the irrigating nozzle. Allow solution to flow out unimpeded.	Solution directed at the roof of the canal aids in preventing injury to the tympanic membrane. Continuous in-and-out flow of the irrigating solution helps prevent pressure in the canal.
When the irrigation is completed, place a cotton ball loosely in the auditory meatus and have the client lie on the side of the affected ear on a towel or an absorbent pad.	The cotton ball absorbs excess fluid. Gravity allows the remaining solution in the canal to escape from the ear.

CHAPTER - 6

DISORDERS OF THE MOUTH

DENTAL CARIES

Dental caries, also known as **tooth decay** or a **cavity**, is an infection, bacterial in origin, that causes demineralization and destruction of the hard tissues of the teeth (enamel, dentin and cementum). It is a result of the production of acid by bacterial fermentation of food debris accumulated on the tooth surface.

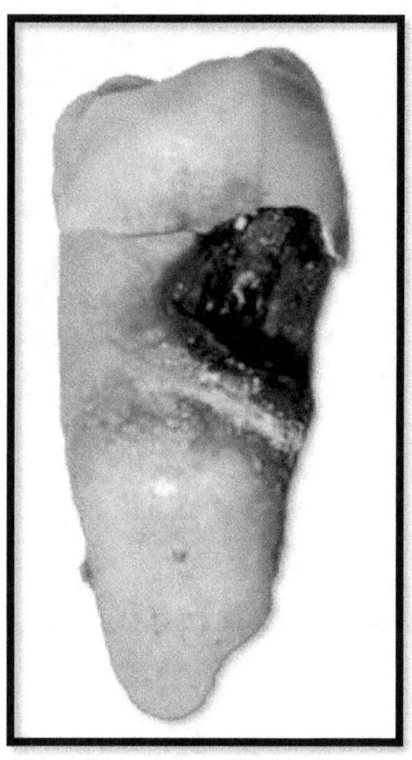

If demineralization exceeds saliva and other remineralization factors such as from calcium and fluoridated toothpastes, these once hard tissues progressively break down, producing dental caries (cavities, holes in the teeth). Today, caries remain one of the most common diseases throughout the world. Cariology is the study of dental caries.

Depending on the extent of tooth destruction, various treatments can be used to restore teeth to proper form, function, and aesthetics, but there is no known method to regenerate large amounts of tooth structure. Instead, dental health

77

organizations advocate preventive and prophylactic measures, such as regular oral hygiene and dietary modifications, to avoid dental caries.

A small spot of decay visible on the surface of a tooth. **(B)** The radiograph reveals an extensive region of demineralization within the dentin (arrows).**(C)** A hole is discovered on the side of the tooth at the beginning of decay removal. **(D)**All decay removed.

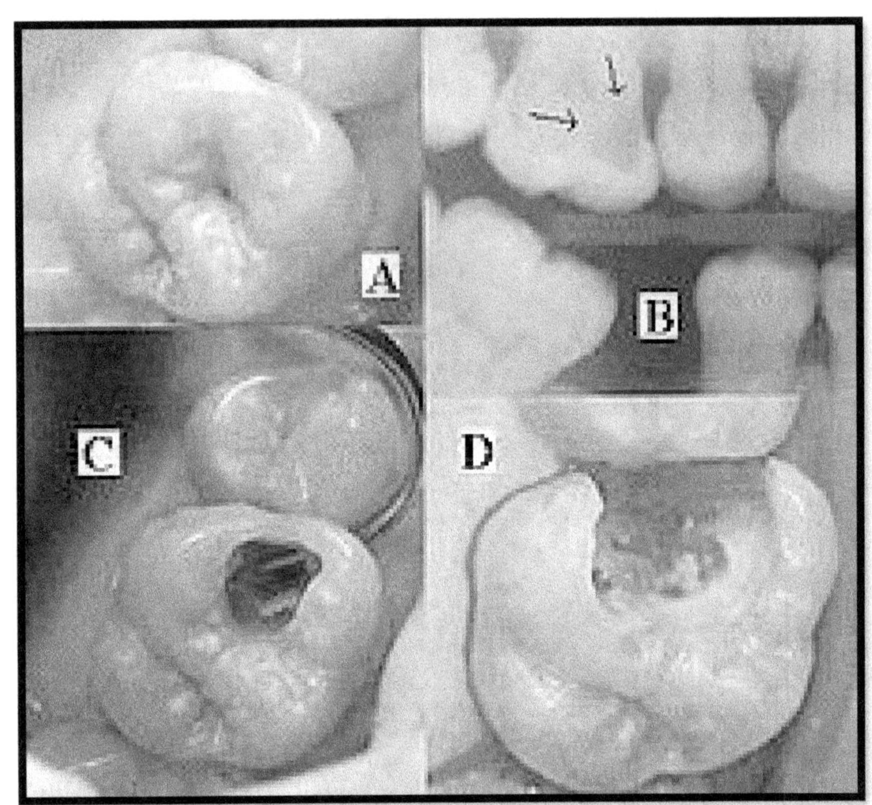

Causes

There are four main criteria required for caries formation: a tooth surface (enamel or dentin); caries-causing bacteria; fermentable carbohydrates (such as sucrose); and time[. The caries process does not have an inevitable outcome, and different individuals will be susceptible to different degrees depending on the shape of their teeth, oral hygiene habits, and the buffering capacity of their saliva. Dental caries can occur on any surface of a tooth that is exposed to the oral cavity, but not the structures that are retained within the bone. The bacteria most responsible for dental cavities are the mutans streptococci, most prominently Streptococcus mutans and Streptococcus sobrinus, and lactobacilli. If left untreated, the diseasecan lead to pain, tooth loss and infection.

Tooth decay disease is caused by specific types of bacteria that produce acid in the presence of fermentable carbohydrates such as sucrose, fructose, and glucose. The mineral content of teeth is sensitive to increases in acidity from the production of lactic acid. To be specific, a tooth (which is primarily mineral in content) is in a constant state of back-and-forth demineralization and remineralization between the tooth and surrounding saliva. For people with little saliva, especially due to radiation therapies and autoimmune disorders, such as Sjögren's syndrome, that may destroy the salivary glands, there also exists therapies such as saliva substitutes and remineralization products. These patients may be susceptible to dental caries. When the pH at the surface of the tooth drops below 5.5, demineralization proceeds faster than remineralization (meaning that there is a net loss of mineral structure on the tooth's surface).

All caries occur from bacterial acid demineralization that exceeds saliva and fluoride remineralization, and acid demineralization occurs where bacterial plaque is left on teeth. Because most plaque-retentive areas are between teeth and inside pits and fissures on chewing surfaces where brushing is difficult, over 80% of cavities occur inside pits and fissures. Areas that are easily cleansed with a toothbrush, such as the front and back surfaces (facial and lingual), develop fewer cavities.

Some foods have an acidic pH of 5.5 or lower which can result in demineralisation in the absence of bacteria. This is known as erosion, rather than caries, because the acid is not bacterial in origin. Attack by acid from systemic complications such as bulimia and stomach difficulties as well as vomiting can cause tooth erosion.

Signs and symptoms

A person experiencing caries may not be aware of the disease. The earliest sign of a new carious lesion is the appearance of a chalky white spot on the surface of the tooth, indicating an area of demineralization of enamel. This is referred to as a white spot lesion, an incipient carious lesion or a "microcavity". As the lesion continues to demineralize, it can turn brown but will eventually turn into a cavitation ("cavity"). Before the cavity forms the process is reversible, but once a cavity forms the lost tooth structure cannot be regenerated. A lesion that appears dark brown and shiny suggests dental caries was once present but the demineralization process has stopped, leaving a stain. Active decay is lighter in color and dull in appearance.

As the enamel and dentin are destroyed, the cavity becomes more noticeable. The affected areas of the tooth change color and become soft to the touch. Once the decay passes through enamel, the dentinal tubules, which have passages to the nerve of the tooth, become exposed, resulting in pain that can be transient, temporarily worsening with exposure to heat, cold, or sweet foods and drinks. A tooth weakened by extensive internal decay can sometimes suddenly fracture under normal chewing forces. When the decay has progressed enough to allow the bacteria to overwhelm the pulp tissue in the center of the tooth a toothache can result and the pain will become more constant. Death of the pulp tissue and infection are common consequences. The tooth will no longer be sensitive to hot or cold, but can be very tender to pressure. Dental caries can also cause bad breath and foul tastes. In highly progressed cases, infection can spread from the tooth to the surrounding soft tissues. Complications such as cavernous sinus thrombosis and Ludwig angina can be life-threatening.

TEETH

There are certain diseases and disorders affecting teeth that may leave an individual at a greater risk for cavities. Amelogenesis imperfecta, which occurs between 1 in 718 and 1 in 14,000 individuals, is a disease in which the enamel does not fully form or forms in insufficient amounts and can fall off a tooth.[16] In both cases, teeth may be left more vulnerable to decay because the enamel is not able to protect the tooth.

In most people, disorders or diseases affecting teeth are not the primary cause of dental caries. Approximately 96% of tooth enamel is composed of minerals. These minerals, especially hydroxyapatite, will become soluble when exposed to acidic

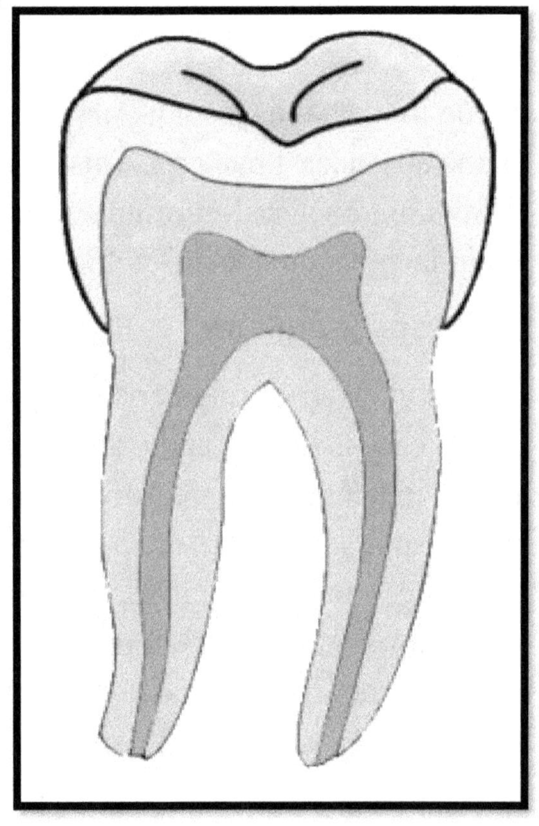

environments. Enamel begins to demineralize at a pH of 5.5. Dentin and cementum are more susceptible to caries than enamel because they have lower mineral content. Thus, when root surfaces of teeth are exposed from gingival recession or periodontal disease, caries can develop more readily. Even in a healthy oral environment, however, the tooth is susceptible to dental caries.

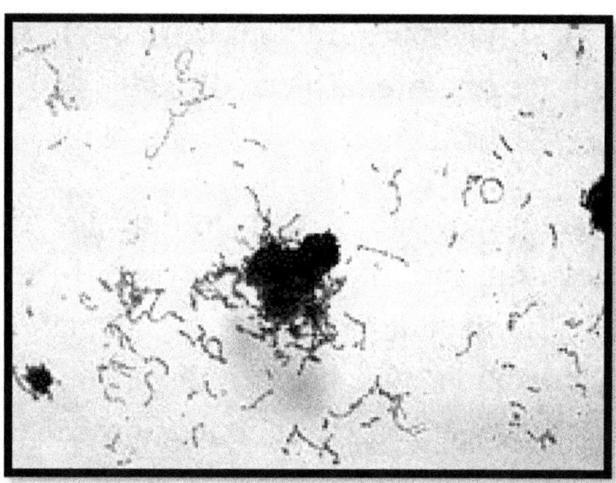

A gram stain image of Streptococcus mutans

The evidence for linking malocclusion and/or crowding to the dental caries is weak; however, the anatomy of teeth may affect the likelihood of caries formation. Where the deep developmental

grooves of teeth are more numerous and exaggerated, pit and fissure caries are more likely to develop (see next section). Also, caries are more likely to develop when food is trapped between teeth.

Bacteria

The mouth contains a wide variety of oral bacteria, but only a few specific species of bacteria are believed to cause dental caries: Streptococcus mutans and Lactobacilli among them. These organisms can produce high levels of lactic acid following fermentation of dietary sugars, and are resistant to the adverse effects of low pH, properties essential for cariogenic bacteria. As the cementum of root surfaces is more easily demineralized than enamel surfaces, a wider variety of bacteria can cause root caries including Lactobacillus acidophilus, Actinomyces spp., Nocardia spp., and Streptococcus mutans. Bacteria collect around the teeth and gums in a sticky, creamy-coloured mass called plaque, which serves as a biofilm. Some sites collect plaque more commonly than others, for example sites with a low rate of salivary flow (molar fissures). Grooves on the occlusal surfaces ofmolar and premolar teeth provide microscopic retention sites for plaque bacteria, as do the interproximal sites. Plaque may also collect above or below the gingiva where it is referred to as supra- or sub-gingival plaque, respectively.

These bacterial strains, most notably S. mutans can be inherited by a child from a caretaker's kiss or through feeding premasticated food.

Fermentable carbohydrates

Bacteria in a person's mouth convert glucose, fructose, and most commonly sucrose (table sugar) into acids such as lactic acid through a glycolytic process called fermentation. If left in contact with the tooth, these acids may cause demineralization, which is the dissolution of its mineral content. The process is dynamic, however, as remineralization can also occur if the acid isneutralized by saliva or mouthwash. Fluoride toothpaste or dental varnish may aid remineralization. If demineralization continues over time, enough mineral content may be lost so that the softorganic material left behind disintegrates, forming a cavity or hole. The impact such sugars have on the progress of dental caries is called cariogenicity. Sucrose, although a bound glucose and fructose unit, is in fact more cariogenic than a mixture of equal parts of glucose and fructose. This is due to the bacteria utilising the energy in the saccharide bond between the glucose and fructose subunits. S.mutans adheres to the biofilm on the tooth by converting sucrose into an extremely adhesive substance called dextran polysaccharide by the enzyme dextransucranase.

Exposure

The frequency of which teeth are exposed to cariogenic (acidic) environments affects the likelihood of caries development. After meals or snacks, the bacteria in the mouth metabolize sugar, resulting in an acidic by-product that decreases pH. As time progresses, the pH returns to normal due to the buffering capacity of saliva and the dissolved mineral content of tooth surfaces. During every exposure to the acidic environment, portions of the inorganic mineral content at the surface of teeth dissolves and can remain dissolved for two hours. Since teeth are vulnerable during these acidic periods, the development of dental caries relies heavily on the frequency of acid exposure.

The carious process can begin within days of a tooth's erupting into the mouth if the diet is sufficiently rich in suitable carbohydrates. Evidence suggests that the introduction of fluoride treatments have slowed the process. Proximal caries take an average of four years to pass through enamel in permanent teeth. Because the cementum enveloping the root surface is not nearly as durable as the enamel encasing the crown, root caries tends to progress much more rapidly than decay on other surfaces. The progression and loss of mineralization on the root surface is 2.5 times faster than caries in enamel. In very severe cases where oral hygiene is very poor and where the diet is very rich in fermentable carbohydrates, caries may cause cavities within months of tooth eruption. This can occur, for example, when children continuously drink sugary drinks from baby bottles (see later discussion).

Other risk factors

Reduced salivary flow rate is associated with increased caries since the buffering capability of saliva is not present to counterbalance the acidic environment created by certain foods. As a result, medical conditions that reduce the amount of saliva produced by salivary glands, in particular the submandibular gland and parotid gland, are likely to dry mouth and thus to widespread tooth decay. Examples include Sjögren's syndrome, diabetes mellitus, diabetes insipidus, and sarcoidosis. Medications, such as antihistamines and antidepressants, can also impair salivary flow. Stimulants, most notoriously methylamphetamine ("meth mouth"), also occlude the flow of saliva to an extreme degree. Tetrahydrocannabinol, the active chemical substance in cannabis, also causes a nearly complete occlusion of salivation, known in colloquial terms as "cotton mouth". Moreover, 63% of the most commonly prescribed medications in the United States list dry mouth as a known side-effect. Radiation therapy of the head and neck may also damage the cells in salivary glands, somewhat increasing the likelihood of caries formation.

The use of tobacco may also increase the risk for caries formation. Some brands of smokeless tobacco contain high sugar content, increasing susceptibility to caries. Tobacco use is a significant risk factor for periodontal disease, which can cause the gingiva to recede. As the gingiva loses attachment to the teeth due to gingival recession, the root surface becomes more visible in the mouth. If this occurs, root caries is a concern since the cementum covering the roots of teeth is more easily demineralized by acids than enamel. Currently, there is not enough evidence to support a causal relationship between smoking and coronal caries, but evidence does suggest a relationship between smoking and root-surface caries.

Intrauterine and neonatal lead exposure promote tooth decay. Besides lead, all atoms with electrical charge and ionic radius similar to bivalent calcium, such ascadmium, mimic the calcium ion and therefore exposure may promote tooth decay. Poverty is also a significant social determinant for oral health. Dental caries have been linked with lower socio-economic status and can be considered a disease of poverty.

Forms are available for risk assessment for caries when treating dental cases; this system using the evidence-based Caries Management by Risk Assessment (CAMBRA). It is still unknown if the identification of high-risk individuals can lead to more effective long-term patient management that prevents caries initiation and arrests or reverses the progression of lesions.

Pathophysiology

Enamel

Enamel is a highly mineralized acellular tissue, and caries act upon it through a chemical process brought on by the acidic environment produced by bacteria. As the bacteria consume the sugar and use it for their own energy, they produce lactic acid. The effects of this process include the demineralization of crystals in the enamel, caused by acids, over time until the bacteria physically penetrate the dentin. Enamel rods, which are the basic unit of the enamel structure, run perpendicularly from the surface of the tooth to the dentin. Since demineralization of enamel by caries, in general, follows the direction of the enamel rods, the different triangular patterns between pit and fissure and smooth-surface caries develop in the enamel because the orientation of enamel rods are different in the two areas of the tooth.

As the enamel loses minerals, and dental caries progresses, the enamel develop several distinct zones, visible under a light microscope. From the deepest layer of the enamel to the enamel surface, the identified areas are the: translucent zone, dark zones, body of the lesion, and surface zone. The translucent zone is the first visible sign of caries and coincides with a one to two percent loss of minerals. A slight remineralization of enamel occurs in the dark zone, which serves as an example of how the development of dental caries is an active process with alternating changes. The area of greatest demineralization and destruction is in the body of the lesion itself. The surface zone remains relatively mineralized and is present until the loss of tooth structure results in a cavitation.

Dentin

Unlike enamel, the dentin reacts to the progression of dental caries. After tooth formation, the ameloblasts, which produce enamel, are destroyed onceenamel formation is complete and thus cannot later regenerate enamel after its destruction. On the other hand, dentin is produced continuously throughout life by odontoblasts, which reside at the border between the pulp and dentin. Since odontoblasts are present, a stimulus, such as caries, can trigger a biologic response. These defense mechanisms include the formation of sclerotic and tertiary dentin.

In dentin from the deepest layer to the enamel, the distinct areas affected by caries are the advancing front, the zone of bacterial penetration, and the zone of destruction. The advancing front represents a zone of demineralised dentine due to acid and has no bacteria present. The zones of bacterial penetration and destruction are the locations of invading bacteria and ultimately the decomposition of dentin. The zone of destruction has a more mixed bacterial population where proteolytic enzymes have destroyed the organic matrix. The innermost dentine caries has been reversibly attacked because the collage matrix is not severely damaged, giving it potential for repair. The outer more superficial zone is highly infected with proteolytic degradation of the collagen matrix and as a result the dentine is irreversibly demineralised.

Sclerotic dentin

The structure of dentin is an arrangement of microscopic channels, called dentinal tubules, which radiate outward from the pulp chamber to the exterior cementum or enamel border. The diameter of the dentinal tubules is largest near the pulp (about 2.5 μm) and smallest (about 900 nm) at the junction of dentin and enamel. The carious process continues through the dentinal tubules, which are responsible for the triangular patterns resulting from the progression of caries deep into the tooth. The tubules also allow caries to progress faster.

In response, the fluid inside the tubules bring immunoglobulins from the immune system to fight the bacterial infection. At the same time, there is an increase of mineralization of the surrounding tubules. This results in a constriction of the tubules, which is an attempt to slow the bacterial progression. In addition, as the acid from the bacteria demineralizes the hydroxyapatite crystals, calcium and phosphorus are released, allowing for the precipitation of more crystals which fall deeper into the dentinal tubule. These crystals form a barrier and slow the advancement of caries. After these protective responses, the dentin is considered sclerotic.

Fluids within dentinal tubules are believed to be the mechanism by which pain receptors are triggered within the pulp of the tooth. Since sclerotic dentin prevents the passage of such fluids, pain that would otherwise serve as a warning of the invading bacteria may not develop at first. Consequently, dental caries may progress for a long period of time without any sensitivity of the tooth, allowing for greater loss of tooth structure.

Tertiary dentin

In response to dental caries, there may be production of more dentin toward the direction of the pulp. This new dentin is referred to as tertiary dentin. Tertiary dentin is produced to protect the pulp for as long as possible from the advancing bacteria. As more tertiary dentin is produced, the size of the pulp decreases. This type of dentin has been subdivided according to the presence or absence of the original odontoblasts. If the odontoblasts survive long enough to react to the dental caries, then the dentin produced is called "reactionary" dentin. If the odontoblasts are killed, the dentin produced is called "reparative" dentin.

In the case of reparative dentin, other cells are needed to assume the role of the destroyed odontoblasts. Growth factors, especially TGF-β, are thought to initiate the production of reparative dentin by fibroblasts and mesenchymal cells of the pulp. Reparative dentin is produced at an average of 1.5 μm/day, but can be increased to 3.5 μm/day. The resulting dentin contains irregularly shaped dentinal tubules that may not line up with existing dentinal tubules. This diminishes the ability for dental caries to progress within the dentinal tubules.

Cementum

The incidence of cemental caries increases in older adults as gingival recession occurs from either trauma or periodontal disease. It is a chronic condition that forms a large, shallow lesion and slowly invades first the root's cementum and then dentin to cause a chronic infection of the pulp (see further discussion under classification by affected hard tissue). Because dental pain is a late finding, many lesions are not detected early, resulting in restorative challenges and increased tooth loss.

Diagnosis:

Adental explorer

The tip of adental explorer, which is used for caries diagnosis.

The presentation of caries is highly variable. However, the risk factors and stages of development are similar. Initially it may appear as a small chalky area (smooth surface caries), which may eventually develop into a large cavitation. Sometimes caries may be directly visible. However other methods of detection such as X-rays are used for less visible areas of teeth and to judge the extent of destruction.

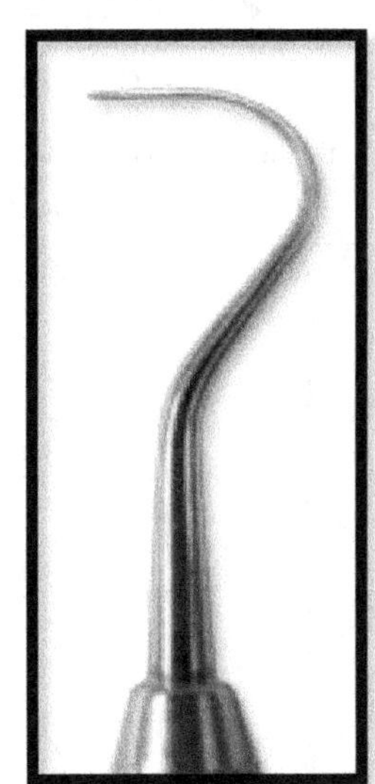

Lasers for detecting caries allow detection without ionizing radiation and are now used for detection of interproximal decay (between the teeth). Disclosing solutions are also used during tooth restoration to minimize the chance of recurrence.

Primary diagnosis involves inspection of all visible tooth surfaces using a good light source, dental mirror and explorer. Dental radiographs (X-rays) may show dental caries before it is otherwise visible, in particular caries between the teeth. Large dental caries is often apparent to the naked eye, but smaller lesions can be difficult to identify. Visual and tactile inspection along with radiographs are employed frequently among dentists, in particular to diagnose pit and fissure caries. Early, uncavitated caries is often diagnosed by blowing air across the suspect surface, which removes moisture and changes the optical properties of the unmineralized enamel.

Some dental researchers have cautioned against the use of dental explorers to find caries. In cases where a small area of tooth has begun demineralizing but has not yet cavitated, the pressure from the dental explorer could cause a cavity. Since the carious process is reversible before a cavity is present, it may be possible to arrest the caries with fluoride and remineralize the tooth surface. When a cavity is present, a restoration will be needed to replace the lost tooth structure.

At times, pit and fissure caries may be difficult to detect. Bacteria can penetrate the enamel to reach dentin, but then the outer surface may remineralize, especially if fluoride is present.[63] These caries, sometimes referred to as "hidden caries", will still be visible on x-ray radiographs, but visual examination of the tooth would show the enamel intact or minimally perforated.

The differential diagnosis for dental caries includes dental fluorosis and developmental defects of the tooth including hypomineralization of the tooth and hypoplasia of the tooth.

Classification

Classification of Restorations

Caries can be classified by location, etiology, rate of progression, and affected hard tissues.[65] These forms of classification can be used to characterize a particular case of tooth decay in order to more accurately represent the condition to others and also indicate the severity of tooth destruction. In some instances, caries are described in other ways that might indicate the cause.

Early childhood caries

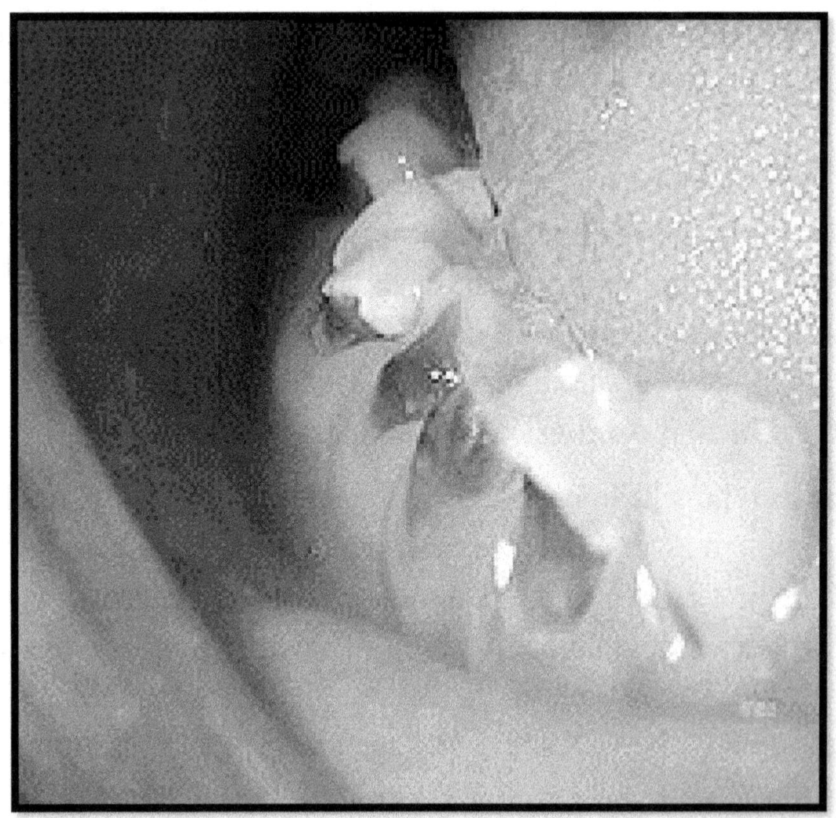

Rampant caries

Early childhood caries (ECC) or "Baby bottle caries," "baby bottle tooth decay," or "Bottle Rot" is a pattern of decay found in young children with theirdeciduous (baby) teeth. The teeth most likely affected are the maxillary anterior teeth, but all teeth can be affected. The name for this type of caries comes from the fact that the decay usually is a result of allowing children to fall asleep with sweetened liquids in their bottles or feeding children sweetened liquids multiple times during the day.

Another pattern of decay is "rampant caries", which signifies advanced or severe decay on multiple surfaces of many teeth. Rampant caries may be seen in individuals with xerostomia, poor oral hygiene, stimulant use (due to drug-induced dry mouth), and/or large sugar intake. If rampant caries is a result of previous radiation to the head and neck, it may be described as radiation-induced caries. Problems can also be caused by the self-destruction of roots and whole tooth resorption when new teeth erupt or later from unknown causes.

Rate of progression

Temporal descriptions can be applied to caries to indicate the progression rate and previous history. "Acute" signifies a quickly developing condition, whereas "chronic" describes a condition that has taken an extended time to develop, in which thousands of meals and snacks, many causing some acid demineralization that is not remineralized, eventually results in cavities.

Recurrent caries, also described as secondary, are caries that appears at a location with a previous history of caries. This is frequently found on the margins of fillings and other dental restorations. On the other hand, incipient caries describes decay at a location that has not experienced previous decay. Arrested caries describes a lesion on a tooth that was previously demineralized but was remineralized before causing a cavitation. Fluoride treatment can help recalcification of tooth enamel as well as use of Amorphous calcium phosphate.

Prevention

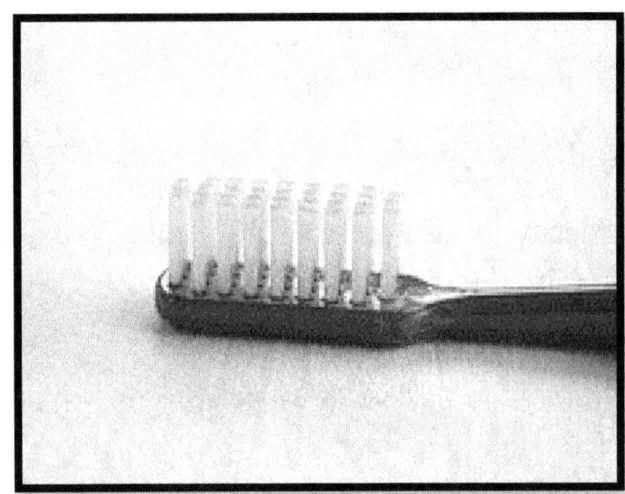

Toothbrushes are commonly used to clean teeth

Oral hygiene

Personal hygiene care consists of proper brushing and flossing daily. The purpose of oral hygiene is to minimize any etiologic agents of disease in the mouth. The primary focus of brushing and flossing is to remove and prevent the formation of plaque or dental biofilm. Plaque consists mostly of bacteria. As the amount of bacterial plaque increases, the tooth is more vulnerable to dental caries when carbohydrates in the food are left on teeth after every meal or snack. A toothbrush can be used to remove plaque on accessible surfaces, but not between teeth or inside pits and fissures on chewing surfaces. When used correctly, dental floss removes plaque from areas that could otherwise develop proximal caries but only if the depth of sulcus has not been compromised. Other adjunct oral hygiene aids include interdental brushes, water picks, and mouthwashes.

However oral hygiene is probably more effective at preventing gum disease (periodontal disease) than tooth decay. Food is forced inside pits and fissures under chewing pressure, leading to carbohydrate-fueled acid demineralisation where the brush, fluoride toothpaste, and saliva have no access to remove trapped food, neutralise acid, or remineralise demineralised tooth like on other more accessible tooth surfaces food to be trapped. (Occlusal caries accounts for between 80 and 90% of caries in children (Weintraub, 2001).) Chewing fibre like celery after eating forces saliva inside trapped food to dilute any carbohydrate like sugar, neutralise acid and remineralise demineralised tooth. The teeth at highest risk for carious lesions are the permanent first and second molars due to length of time in oral cavity and presence of complex surface anatomy.

Professional hygiene care consists of regular dental examinations and professional prophylaxis (cleaning). Sometimes, complete plaque removal is difficult, and a dentist or dental hygienist may be needed. Along with oral hygiene, radiographs may be taken at dental visits to detect possible dental caries development in high risk areas of the mouth, along with compliance to strict radiographic guidelines established by dental associations such as the American Dental Association and American Dental Hygienists' Association.

Dietary modification

For dental health, frequency of sugar intake is more important than the amount of sugar consumed.

In the presence of sugar and other carbohydrates, bacteria in the mouth produce acids that can demineralize enamel, dentin, and cementum. The more frequently teeth are exposed to this environment the more likely dental caries are to occur. Therefore, minimizing snacking is recommended, since snacking creates a continuous supply of nutrition for acid-creating bacteria in the mouth. Also, chewy and sticky foods (such as dried fruit or candy) tend to adhere to teeth longer, and, as a consequence, are best eaten as part of a meal. Brushing the teeth after meals is recommended. For children, the American Dental Association and the European Academy of Paediatric Dentistry recommend limiting the frequency of consumption of drinks with sugar, and not giving baby bottles to infants during sleep (see earlier discussion).

Mothers are also recommended to avoid sharing utensils and cups with their infants to prevent transferring bacteria from the mother's mouth.

It has been found that milk and certain kinds of cheese like cheddar cheese can help counter tooth decay if eaten soon after the consumption of foods potentially harmful to teeth. Also, chewing containing xylitol (a sugar alcohol) is widely used to protect teeth in many countries now. Xylitol's effect on reducing dental biofilm is, it is presumed, due to bacteria's inability to utilize it like other sugars. Chewing and stimulation of flavour receptors on the tongue are also known to increase the production and release of saliva, which contains natural buffers to prevent the lowering of pH in the mouth to the point where enamel may become demineralized.

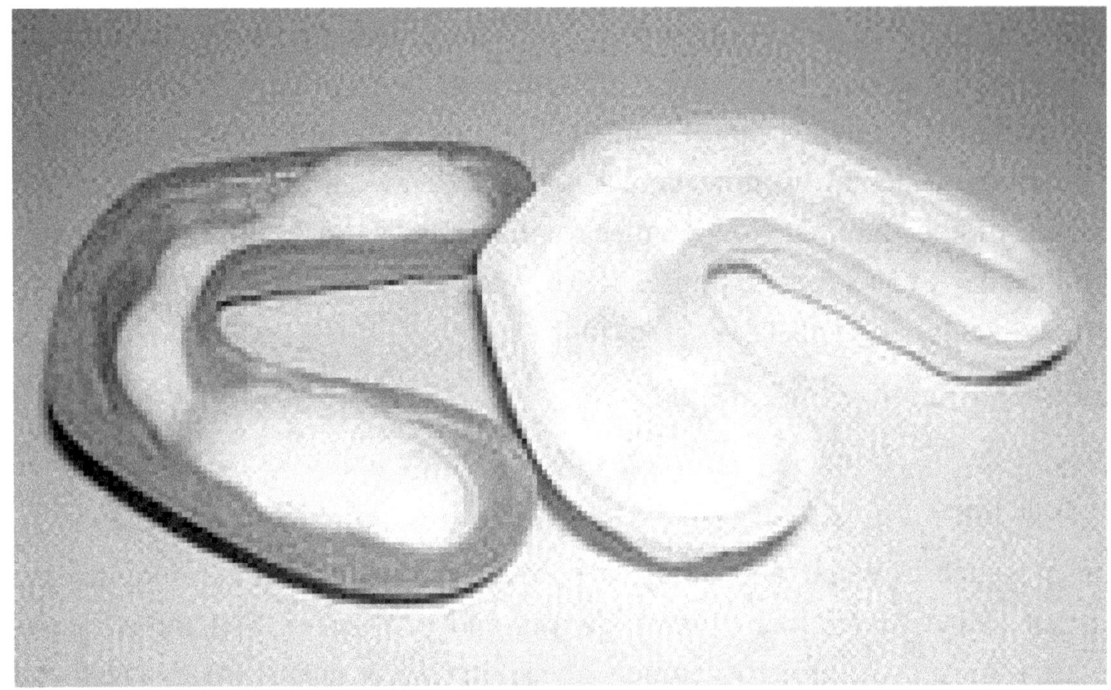

Common dentistry trays used to deliver fluoride

Other measures

The use of dental sealants is a means of prevention. A sealant is a thin plastic-like coating applied to the chewing surfaces of the molars to prevent food from being trapped inside pits and fissures. This deprives resident plaque bacteria carbohydrate preventing the formation of pit and fissure caries. Sealants are usually applied on the teeth of children, as soon as the tooth erupt but adults are receiving them if not previously performed. Sealants can wear out and fail to prevent access of food and plaque bacteria inside pits and fissures and need to be replaced so they must be checked regularly by dental professionals.

Calcium, as found in food such as milk and green vegetables, is often recommended to protect against dental caries. Fluoride helps prevent decay of a tooth by binding to the hydroxyapatite crystals in enamel. The incorporated calcium makes enamel more resistant to demineralization and, thus, resistant to decay. Topical fluoride is now more highly recommended than systemic intake such as by tablets or drops to protect the surface of the teeth. This may include a fluoride toothpaste or mouthwash or varnish. Many dental professionals include application of topical fluoride solutions as part of routine visits and recommend the use of xylitol and Amorphous calcium phosphate products.

Vaccines are also under development.

Treatment

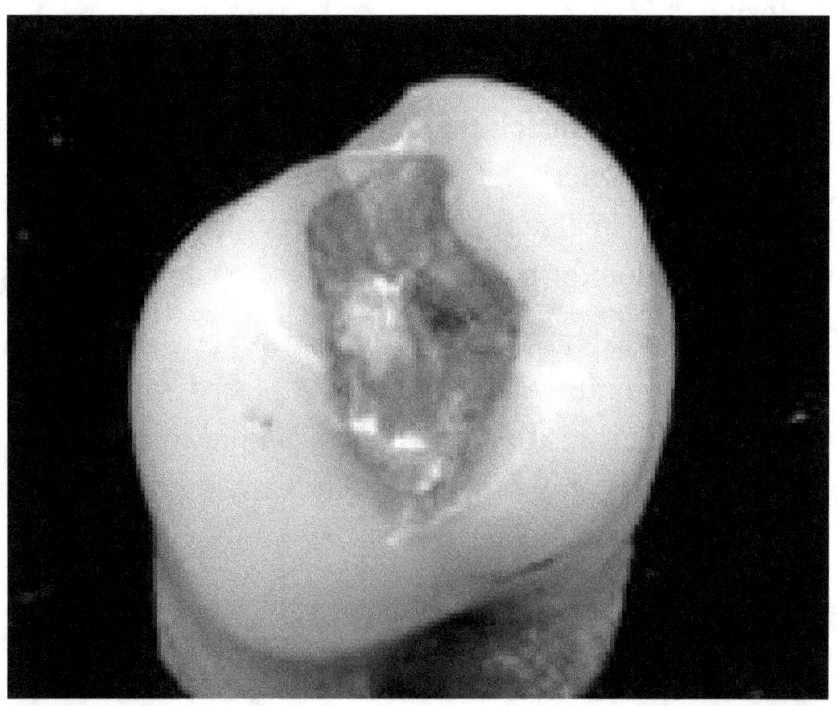

An amalgam used as a restorative material in a tooth

Destroyed tooth structure does not fully regenerate, although remineralization of very small carious lesions may occur if dental hygiene is kept at optimal level. For the small lesions, topical fluoride is sometimes used to encourage remineralization. For larger lesions, the progression of dental caries can be stopped by treatment. The goal of treatment is to preserve tooth structures and prevent further destruction of the tooth. Aggressive treatment, by filling, of incipient carious lesions, places where there is superficial damage to the enamel, is controversial as they may heal themselves, while once a filling is performed it will eventually have to be redone and the site serves as a vulnerable site for further decay.

In general, early treatment is less painful and less expensive than treatment of extensive decay. Anesthetics—local, nitrous oxide ("laughing gas"), or other prescription medications—may be required in some cases to relieve pain during or following treatment or to relieve anxiety during treatment. A dental handpiece ("drill") is used to remove large portions of decayed material from a tooth. A spoon, a dental instrument used to carefully remove decay, is sometimes employed when the decay in dentin reaches near the pulp. Once the decay is removed, the missing tooth structure requires a dental restoration of some sort to return the tooth to function and aesthetic condition.

Restorative materials

It includes dental amalgam, composite resin, porcelain, and gold. Composite resin and porcelain can be made to match the colour of a patient's natural teeth and are thus used more frequently when aesthetics are a concern. Composite restorations are not as strong as dental amalgam and gold; some dentists consider the latter as the only advisable restoration for posterior areas where chewing forces are great.

When the decay is too extensive, there may not be enough tooth structure remaining to allow a restorative material to be placed within the tooth. Thus, a crown may be needed. This restoration appears similar to a cap and is fitted over the remainder of the natural crown of the tooth. Crowns are often made of gold, porcelain, or porcelain fused to metal.

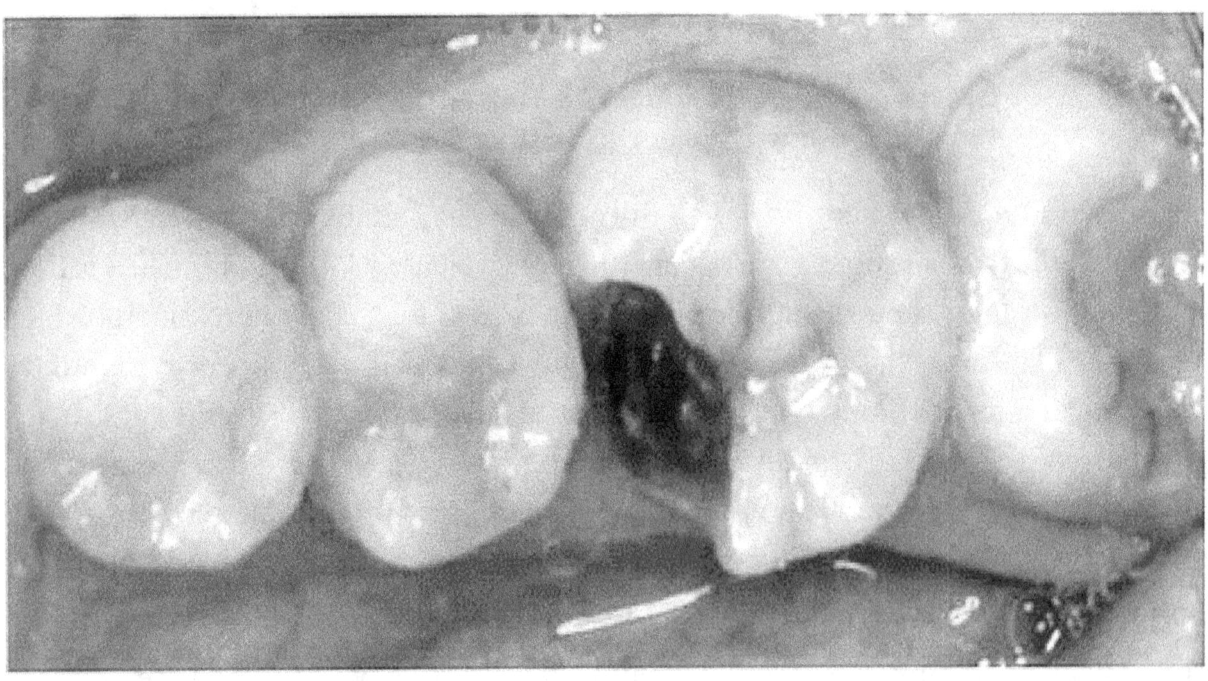

A tooth with extensive caries

Extraction

In certain cases, endodontic therapy may be necessary for the restoration of a tooth. Endodontic therapy, also known as a "root canal", is recommended if the pulp in a tooth dies from infection by decay-causing bacteria or from trauma. During a root canal, the pulp of the tooth, including the nerve and vascular tissues, is removed along with decayed portions of the tooth. The canals are instrumented with endodontic files to clean and shape them, and they are then usually filled with a rubber-like material called gutta percha. The tooth is filled and a crown can be placed. Upon completion of a root canal, the tooth is now non-vital, as it is devoid of any living tissue.

An extraction can also serve as treatment for dental caries. The removal of the decayed tooth is performed if the tooth is too far destroyed from the decay process to effectively restore the tooth. Extractions are sometimes considered if the tooth lacks an opposing tooth or will probably cause further problems in the future, as may be the case for wisdom teeth. Extractions may also be preferred by patients unable or unwilling to undergo the expense or difficulties in restoring the tooth.

PERIODONTAL DISEASE

Periodontal disease is a type of disease that affects one or more of the periodontal tissues:

1. Alveolar Bone
2. Periodontal Ligament
3. Cementum
4. Gingiva

While many different diseases affect the tooth-supporting structures, plaque-induced inflammatory lesions make up the vast majority of periodontal diseases and have traditionally been divided into two categories:

1. Gingivitis
2. Periodontitis.

Diagnosis

In 1976, Page & Schroeder introduced an innovative new analysis of periodontal disease based on histopathologic and ultrastructural features of the diseased gingival tissue. Although this new classification does not correlate with clinical signs and symptoms and is admittedly "somewhat arbitrary," it permits a focus of attention pathologic aspects of the disease that were, until recently, not well understood.

This new classification divided plaque-induced periodontal lesions into four stages:

1. Initial Lesion
2. Early Lesion
3. Established Lesion
4. Advanced Lesion

Initial lesion

Unlike most regions of the body, the oral cavity is perpetually populated by pathogenic microorganisms; because there is a constant challenge to the mucosa in the form of these microorganisms and their harmful products, it is difficult to truly characterize the boundary between health and disease activity in the periodontal tissues. The oral cavity contains over 500 different microorganisms. It is very hard to distinguish exactly which periodontal pathogen is causing the breakdown of tissues and bone. As such, the initial lesion is said to merely reflect "enhanced levels of activity" of host response mechanisms "normally operative within the gingival tissues."

Healthy gingiva are characterized by small numbers of leukocytes migrating towards the gingival sulcus and residing in the junctional epithelium. Sparse lymphocytes, and plasma cells in particular, may exist just after exiting small blood vessels deep within the underlying connective tissue of the soft tissue between teeth. There is, however, no tissue damage, and the presence of such cells is not considered to be an indication of a pathologic change. When looking at the gums they look knife like and a very light pink or coral pink.

On the contrary, the initial lesion shows increased capillary permeability with "very large numbers" of neutrophils migrating from the dilated gingival plexus into the junctional epithelium and underlying connective tissue (yet remaining within the confines of the region of the sulcus) and macrophages and lymphocytes may also appear. Loss of perivascular collagen occurs; it is thought that this is due to the degradative enzymes released by extravasating leukocytes, such that the collagen and other connective tissue fibres surrounding blood vessels in the area dissolve. When this occurs, the gums will appear bright red and either bulbous or rounded, from all the excess fluid building up in the infected area.

The initial lesion appears within two to four days of gingival tissue being subjected to plaque accumulation. When not generated through clinical experimentation, the initial lesion may not appear at all, and instead, a detectable infiltrate similar to that of the early lesion, explained below, appears.

Features of the Initial Lesion

- Vasculitis of vessels subjacent to junctional epithelium
- Increased migration of leukocytes into junctional epithelium
- Extravascular presence of serum proteins, especially fibrin
- Alteration of the most coronal portion of junctional epithelium
- Loss of perivascular collagen

Early lesion

While the early lesion is not entirely distinct from the initial lesion, it is said to encompass the inflammatory changes that occur from days four to seven after plaque accumulation has commenced. It is characterized by a matured leukocytic infiltrate that feature mainly lymphocytes. Immunoblasts are quite common in the area of infiltration, while plasma cells, if present, are only at the edges of the area. The early lesion can occupy up to 15% of the connective tissue of the marginal gingiva and up to 60-70% of collagen may be dissolved.

Fibroblasts appear altered, exhibiting electron-lucent nuclei, swollen mitochondria, vacuolization of the rough endoplasmic reticulum and rupture of their cell membranes, appearing up to three times the size of normal fibroblasts and found in association with moderately-sized lymphocytes.

The early lesion displays acute exudative inflammation; exudative components and crevicular lymphocytes reach their maximum levels between days 6-12 after plaque accumulates and gingival inflammation commences with the quantity of crevicular fluid being proportional to the size of the reaction site within the underlying connective tissue. The junctional epithelium may even become infiltrated with enough leukocytes so that it resembles a micro abscess.

Features of the Early Lesion

➢ Accentuation of features of the initial lesion, such as the considerably greater loss of collagen
➢ Accumulation of lymphocytes subjacent to junctional epithelium
➢ Cytopathic alterations in resident fibroblasts
➢ Preliminary proliferation of basal cells of junctional epithelium

Established lesion

The hallmark of the established lesion if the overwhelming presence of plasma cells in relation to the prior stages of inflammation. Beginning two to three weeks after first plaque formation, the established lesion is widespread in both human and animals populations and can be seen commonly associated with the placement of orthodontic bands on molars.

Similar to the initial and early lesions, the established lesion features an inflammatory reaction confined to the area near the base of the gingival sulcus, but unlike prior stages, displays plasma cells clustered around blood vessels and between collagen fibres outside the immediate area of the reaction site. While most of the plasma cells produce IgG, a significant number do produce IgA (and rarely, some produce IgM). The presence of complement and antigen-antibody complexes is evident throughout the connective and epithelial tissue.

It is in the established lesion that epithelial proliferation and apical migration begin. In health, the junctional epithelium creates the most coronal attachment of the gum tissue to the tooth at or near the cementoenamel junction. In the established lesion of periodontal disease, the connective tissue lying subjacent to the junctional epithelium is nearly destroyed, failing to properly support the epithelium and buttress it against the tooth surface.

In response to this, the junctional epithelium proliferates and grows into the vacant underlying spaces, effectively causing the level of its attachment to migrate towards apically, revealing more tooth structure than is normally evident supragingivally (above the level of the gumline) in health.

While many established lesions continue to the advanced lesion (below), most either remain as established lesions for decades or indefinitely; the mechanisms behind this phenomenon are not well understood.

Features of the Established Lesion

- Predominance of plasma cells without bone loss
- Presence of extravascular immunoglobulins in the connective tissue and junctional epithelium
- Continuing loss of collagen
- Proliferation, apical migration and lateral extension of the junctional epithelium, with or without pocket formation

Advanced lesion

- Many of the features of the advanced lesion are Periodontal pocket formation
- Gingival ulceration and suppuration
- Destruction of the alveolar bone and periodontal ligament
- Tooth mobility, drifting and eventual loss

Described clinically rather than histologically

Because bone loss makes its first appearance in the advanced lesion, it is equated with periodontitis, while the first three lesions are classified as gingivitis in levels of increasing severity. The advanced lesion is no longer localized to the area around the gingival sulcus but spreads apically as well as laterally around a tooth and perhaps even deep into the gum tissue papilla. There is a dense infiltrate of plasma cells, other lymphocytes and macrophages. The clusters of perivascular plasma cells still appear from the established lesion. Bone is resorbed, producing scarring and fibrous change.

Features of the Advanced Lesion

- Extension of the lesion into alveolar bone, periodontal ligament with significant bone loss
- Continued loss of collagen
- Cytopathic alterations in plasma cells in the absence of altered fibroblasts
- Formation of periodontal pocketing
- Conversion of bone marrow into fibrous connective tissue

Treatment

The treatment of periodontal disease begins with the removal of sub-gingival calculus (tartar) and biofilm deposits. A dental hygienist procedure called scaling and root planning is the common first step in addressing periodontal problems, which seeks to remove calculus by mechanically scraping it from tooth surfaces.

Dental calculus, commonly known as tartar, consists almost entirely of calcium phosphate salt, the ionic derivative of calcium phosphate (the primary composition of teeth and bone). Dental calculus deposits harbour harmful bacteria. Clinically, calculus stuck to teeth appears to be hardened to the point requiring mechanical scraping for removal.

The bacteria responsible for most periodontal disease is anaerobic, and oxygenation reduces populations. Thorough brushing with dilute hydrogen peroxide, with emphasis on the gum line, and flossing, help prevent the formation of harmful biofilm, gingivitis, and tartar. Therapeutic mechanical delivery of hydrogen peroxide to sub gingival pockets can be provided by a water pick. Wound "healing following gingival surgery was enhanced due to the antimicrobial effects of topically administered hydrogen peroxide". For most subjects, beneficial effects were seen with hydrogen peroxide levels above 1% though concentrations between 1% and 3% have been suggested, and commercial preparations contain 1.5% hydrogen peroxide. Enzymatic agents found in commercial preparations can loosen, dissolve, and prevent biofilm formation. Beneficial agents include lysozyme, lactoperozidase, glucose oxidase, mutanase, and dextranase. Another method for treatment of periodontal disease involve the use of an orally administered antibiotic, Periostat (Doxycycline). Periostat has been clinically proven to decrease alveolar bone loss and improve the conditions of periodontal disease with minimal side-effects. However, Periostat does not kill the bacteria, as it only inhibits the body's host response to destroy the tissue.

Laser-assisted periodontal therapy has been shown to kill the bacteria that causes periodontal disease as well as grow bone in certain cases.

Prognosis

Plaque, also known as a biofilm, when examined under a microscope, is made of millions (10^6-8) of bacteria. There are many different types of microbes contained in the biofilm of those with periodontal disease. Two major bacteria implicated are "Porphyromonas gingivalis" and "Aggregatibacter actinomycetemcomitans" A. actinomycetemcomitans is associated with acquired resistance to normal treatments against periodontal disease. P. gingivalis can produce harmful enzymes which disrupt the host immune system and lead to massive tissue destruction. Since a microbe is a living organism, it maintains some of the same properties that we do to survive. Porphyromonas have a life cycle, they have a digestive system, and they reproduce. Bacteria have to eat to survive; they also have to eliminate wastes and are constantly reproducing. Naturally, bacteria are always present in the oral cavity. However, when plaque is not removed on a daily basis, trouble begins.

Bacteria around teeth cause the destruction and foul odors in a person with gum disease, specifically sulfur-containing compounds. Bone is considered to be the foundation and supporting structure of teeth. Bacteria will make themselves at home in the spaces between teeth and release or exhibit compounds that the body's immune response leads to inflammation resulting in bone loss. As bacteria proliferate, the immune response increases and teeth will eventually become loose and either fall out on their own, or are extracted by a dentist. This process is not something that happens overnight.

It is recommended that a dental prophylaxis and thorough examination of the mouth be done every six months, preventing plaque build-up on teeth. Plaque or bacteria, if left for a long period of time, eventually die off. Dead plaque hardens and calcifies and is then referred to as tartar, or calculus. Once the calculus builds up around the teeth, in between them, and the gums, it causes the gums to pull away from the teeth. When the gums pull away from the teeth, a pocket is created which allows food and debris to accumulate, harbouring even more bacteria. This also allows bacteria to enter the bloodstream. Studies have shown that heart disease is almost twice as likely to occur in people with gum disease. Studies have also shown that the most common strain of bacteria found in dental plaque may cause blood clots. When blood clots escape into the bloodstream, there is a relation to increased risk of heart attacks, and other illnesses.

TOOTH ABSCESS

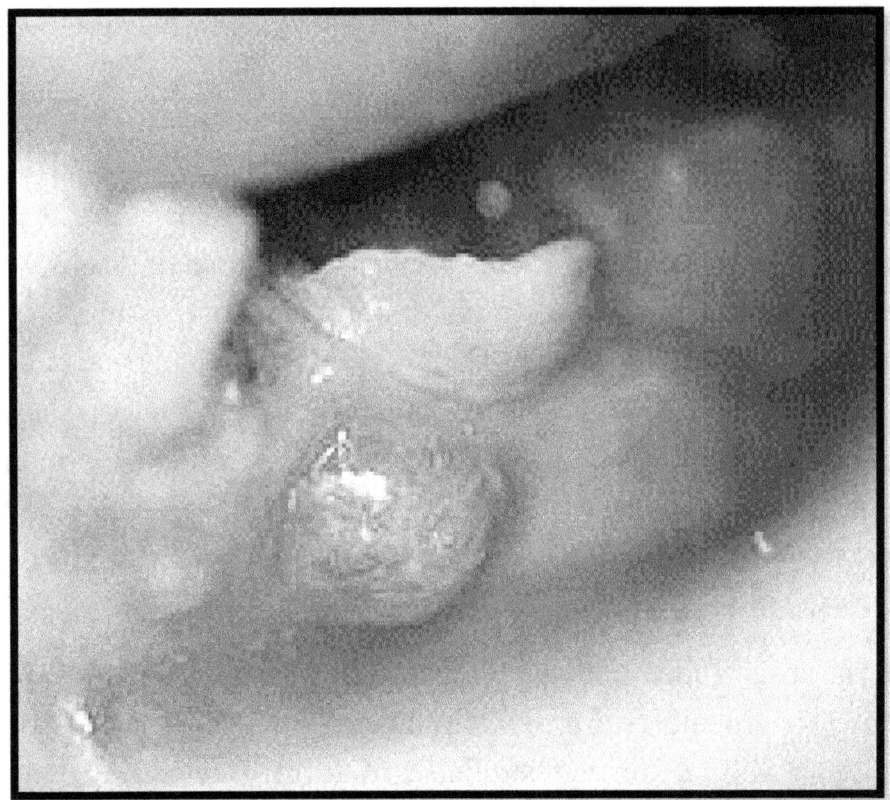

A decayed and broken down tooth, which has undergone pulpal necrosis (death of the tooth pulp). A periapical abscess (i.e. around the apex of the tooth root) has then formed and pus is draining into the mouth via an intra-oral sinus (colloquially termed agumboil).

A **tooth abscess** or **root abscess** is pus enclosed in the tissues of the jaw bone at the apex of an infected tooth's root(s). Usually the abscess originates from a bacterial infection that has accumulated in the soft, often dead, pulp of the tooth. This can be caused by tooth decay, broken teeth or extensive periodontal disease (or combinations of these factors). A failed root canal treatment may also create a similar abscess.

Examples of types of dental abscess include

- Gingival abscesses: involves only the gum tissue, without affecting either the tooth or the periodontal ligament.
- Periapical abscesses: starts at the apex of the root.
- Periodontal abscesses: begin in the pocket of gingiva over 3 mm.

Signs and symptoms

The pain is continuous and may be described as extreme, gnawing, sharp, shooting, or throbbing. Putting pressure or warmth on the tooth may induce extreme pain. There may be a swelling present at either the base of the tooth, the gum, and/or the cheek, which can be reduced by applying ice packs. An acute abscess may be painless but still have a swelling present on the gum. It is important to get anything that presents like this checked by a dental professional as it may become chronic later.

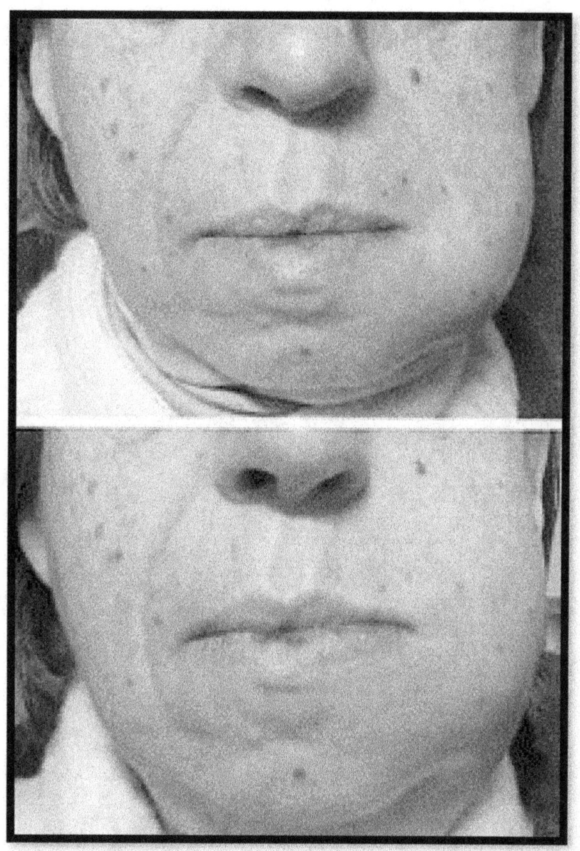

An abscess originating from a tooth (buccal space). Above, deformation of the cheek on the second day. Below, deformation on the third day

In some cases, a tooth abscess may perforate bone and start draining into the surrounding tissues creating local facial swelling. In some cases, the lymph glands in the neck will become swollen and tender in response to the infection. It may even feel like a migraine as the pain can transfer from the infected area. The pain does not normally transfer across the face, only upwards or downwards as the nerves that serve each side of the face are separate.

Severe aching and discomfort on the side of the face where the tooth is infected is also fairly common, with the tooth itself becoming unbearable to touch due to extreme amounts of pain.

Treatment

dental abscess centres on the reduction and elimination of the offending organisms. This can include treatment with antibiotics and drainage. If the tooth can be restored, root canal therapy can be performed. Non-restorable teeth must be extracted, followed by curettage of all apical soft tissue.

Unless they are symptomatic, teeth treated with root canal therapy should be evaluated at 1- and 2-years intervals to rule out possible lesional enlargement and to ensure appropriate healing.

Abscesses may fail to heal for several reasons

- Cyst formation
- Inadequate root canal therapy
- Vertical root fractures
- Foreign material in the lesion
- Associated periodontal disease
- Penetration of the maxillary sinus

Following conventional, adequate root canal therapy, abscesses that do not heal or enlarge are often treated with surgery and filling the root tips; and will require a biopsy to evaluate the diagnosis.

Complications if untreated

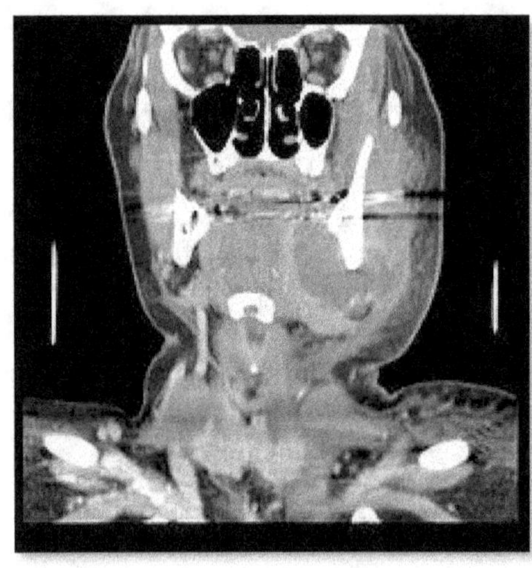

CT scan showing a large tooth abscess (right in the image) with significant inflammation of fatty tissue under the skin

If left untreated, a severe tooth abscess may become large enough to perforate bone and extend into the soft tissue eventually becoming osteomyelitis and cellulitis respectively. From there it follows the path of least resistance and may spread either internally or externally. The path of the infection is influenced by such things as the location of the infected tooth and the thickness of the bone, muscle and fascia attachments.

External drainage may begin as a boil which bursts allowing pus drainage from the abscess, intraorally (usually through the gum) or extra orally. Chronic drainage will allow an epithelial lining to form in this communication to form a pus draining canal (fistula). Sometimes this type of drainage will immediately relieve some of the painful symptoms associated with the pressure.

Internal drainage is of more concern as growing infection makes space within the tissues surrounding the infection. Severe complications requiring immediate hospitalization include Ludwig's angina, which is a combination of growing infection and cellulitis which closes the airway space causing suffocation in extreme cases. Also infection can spread down the tissue spaces to the mediastinum which has significant consequences on the vital organs such as the heart. Another complication, usually from upper teeth, is a risk of septicaemia (infection of the blood) from connecting into blood vessels, brain abscess (extremely rare), or meningitis (also rare).

STOMATITIS

Stomatitis is inflammation in the mouth. The term refers to any inflammatory process affecting the mucous membranes of the mouth and lips, with or without oral ulceration. The inflammation can be caused by conditions in the mouth itself, such as poor oral hygiene, dietary protein deficiency, poorly fitted dentures, or from mouth burns and scars from food or drinks, toxic plants, or by conditions that affect the entire body, such as medications, allergic reactions, radiation therapy, or infections.

Severe iron deficiency anaemia can lead to stomatitis. Iron is necessary for the upregulation of transcriptional elements for cell replication and repair. Lack of iron can cause the genetic downregulation of these elements, leading to ineffective repair and regeneration of epithelial cells, especially in the mouth and lips. This condition is also prevalent in people who have a deficiency in vitamin B_2 (Riboflavin), B_3 (Niacin), B_6 (Pyridoxine), B_9 (folic acid) or B_{12} (cobalamine).

When it also involves an inflammation of the gingiva (gums), it is called.

It may also be seen in ariboflavinosis (riboflavin deficiency) or neutropenia.

Classification

Aphthous stomatitis

Aphthous stomatitis (canker sores) is the recurrent appearance of mouth ulcers in otherwise healthy individuals. The cause is not completely understood, but it is thought that the condition represents an T cell mediated immune response which is triggered by a variety of factors. The individual ulcers (aphthae) recur periodically and heal completely, although in the more severe forms new ulcers may appear in other parts of the mouth before the old ones have finished healing. Aphthous stomatitis is one of the most common diseases of the oral mucosa, and is thought to affect about 20% of the general population to some degree. The symptoms range from a minor nuisance to being disabling in their impact on eating, swallowing and talking, and the severe forms can cause people to loose weight. There is no cure for aphthous stomatitis, and therapies are aimed at alleviating the pain, reducing the inflammation and promoting healing of the ulcers, but there is little evidence of efficacy for any treatment that has been used.

Angular stomatitis

Inflammation of the corners (angles) of the lips is termed angular stomatitis or angular cheilitis. In children a frequent cause is repeated lip-licking and in adults it may be a sign of underlying iron deficiency anaemia, or vitamin B deficiencies (e.g. B_2-riboflavin, B_9-folate or B_{12}-cobalamin, which in turn may be evidence of poor diets or malnutrition such as celiac disease).

Also, angular cheilitis can be caused by a patient's jaws at rest being 'over closed' due to edentulousness or tooth wear, causing the jaws to come to rest closer together than if the complete/unaffected dentition were present. This causes skin folds around the angle of the mouth which are kept moist by saliva which in turn favours infection; mostly by Candida albicans or similar species. Treatment usually involves the administration of topical nystatin or similar antifungal agents. Another treatment can be to correct the jaw relationship with dental treatment (e.g. dentures or occlusal adjustment).

Denture-related stomatitis

This is a common condition present in denture wearers. It appears as reddened but painless mucosa beneath the denture. 90% of cases are associated with Candidia species, and it is the most common form of oral candidiasis. Treatment is by antifungal medication and improved dental hygiene, such as not wearing the denture during sleep.

Migratory stomatitis

Migratory stomatitis (or geographic stomatitis) is an atypical presentation of a condition which normally presents on the tongue, termed geographic tongue. Geographic tongue is so named because there are atrophic, erythematous areas of depapillation that migrate over time, giving a map-like appearance. In migratory stomatitis, other mucosal sites in the mouth, such as the ventral surface (undersurface) of the tongue, buccal mucosa, labial mucosa, soft palate or floor of mouth may be afflicted with identical lesions, usually in addition to the tongue. Apart from not being restricted to the tongue, migratory stomatitis is an identical condition in every regard to geographic tongue. Another synonym for geographic tongue which uses the term stomatitis is "stomatitis areata migrans".

Stomatitis Nicotina

Chronic ulcerative stomatitis

Chronic ulcerative stomatitis is a recently discovered condition with specific immunopathologic features. It is characterized by erosions and ulcerations which relapse and remit. Lesions are located on the buccal mucosa (inside of the cheeks) or on the gingiva (gums). It is characterized by painful erosions and ulcerations which relapse and remit. This condition resembles Oral lichen planus when biopsied. The diagnosis is made with Immunofluorescence techniques, which shows circulating and tissue-bound autoantibodies (particulate stratified squamous-epithelium-specific antinuclear antibody) to DeltaNp63alpha protein, a normal component of the epithelium. Treatment is with hydroxychloroquine.

Other forms of stomatitis

o Periodic fever, aphthous stomatitis, pharyngitis and adenitis (PFAPA) syndrome-- occurs in children.
o Uremic stomatitis-- a rare form of stomatitis that occurs with renal failure.

ORAL THRUSH OR MONILIASIS

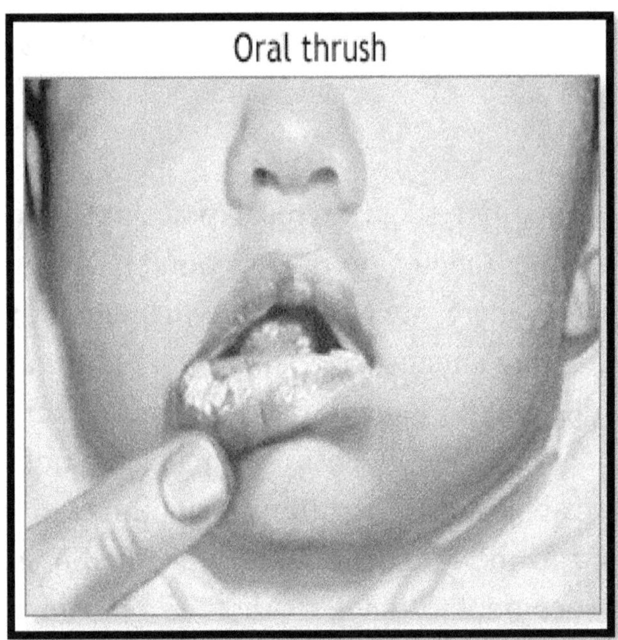

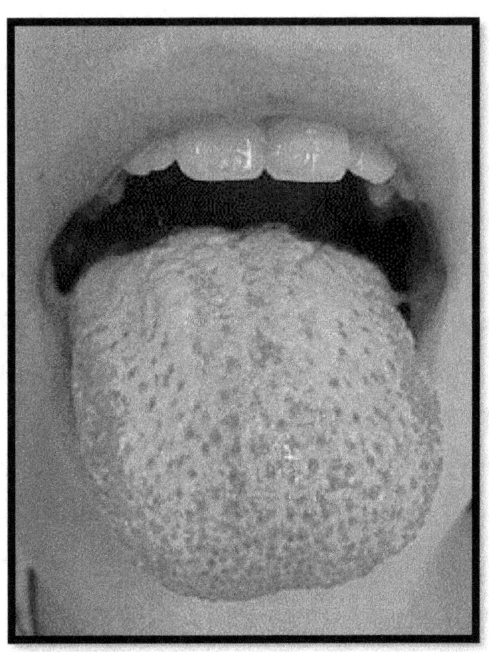

Oral candidiasis (also known as **oral candidosis, oral thrush, oropharyngeal candidiasis, moniliasis, candidal stomatitis, muguet**) iscandidiasis occurring in the mouth. That is, oral candidiasis is a mycosis (yeast/fungal infection) of Candida species on the mucous membranes of the mouth.

Causes

Candida albicans is the most commonly implicated organism in this condition. C. albicans is carried in the mouths of about 50% of the world's population as a normal component of the oral microbiota. This candidal carriage state is not considered a disease, but when candida species become pathogenic and invade host tissues, oral candidiasis can occur. This change usually constitutes an opportunistic infection of normally harmless micro-organisms because of local (i.e. mucosal), or systemic factors altering host immunity.

Classification

<table>
<tr><td colspan="1">Traditional classification of oral candidiasis</td></tr>
</table>

- **Acute candidiasis:**
  - pseudomembranous candidiasis (oral thrush)
  - atrophic candidiasis
- **Chronic candidiasis:**
  - atrophic candidiasis
  - hyperplastic candidiasis
  - chronic oral candidiasis (Candida leukoplakia)
  - candidiasis endocrinopathy syndrome
  - chronic localized mucocutaneous candidiasis
  - chronic diffuse candidiasis.

<table>
<tr><td colspan="1">Classification of oral candidiasis</td></tr>
</table>

- **Primary oral candidiasis (group I)**
  - Pseudomembranous (acute or chronic)
  - Erythematous (acute or chronic)
  - Hyperplastic: plaque-like, nodular
  - Candida-associated lesions: Denture related stomatitis, angular stomatitis, median rhomboid glossitis, linear gingival erythema
- **Secondary oral candidiasis (group II)**
  - Oral manifestations of systemic mucocutaneous candidiasis (due to diseases such as thymic aplasia and candidiasis endocrinopathy syndrome)

Being a type of candidiasis, oral candidiasis is a mycosis. Traditionally, oral candidiasis is classified using the Lehner system, originally described in the 1960s, into acute and chronic forms. The fact that some of the subtypes traditionally almost always either acute or chronic (e.g. acute pseudomembranous candidiasis) occasionally may present as either acute or chronic created problems with this system. The global human immunodeficiency virus/acquired immunodeficiency syndrome (HIV/AIDS) pandemic has been an important factor in this change. A more recently proposed classification of oral candidiasis distinguishes primary oral candidiasis, where the condition is confined to the mouth and perioral tissues, andsecondary oral candidiasis, where there is involvement of other parts of the body in addition to the mouth.

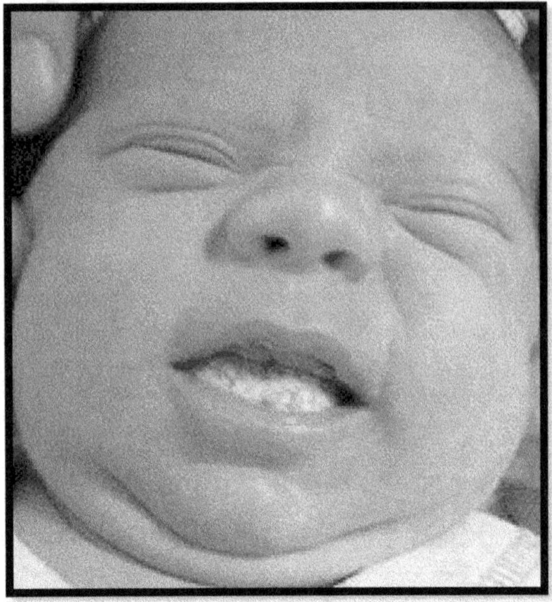

Oral candidiasis in an infant. At very young ages, the immune system is yet to develop fully.

Oropharyngeal candidiasis, pseudomembranous type

By clinical appearance

Three main clinical appearances of candidiasis are generally recognized: pseudomembranous, erythematous (atrophic) and hyperplastic. Most often individuals affected will display one clear type or another, but sometimes there can be more than one clinical variant in the same person.

Pseudomembranous

Acute pseudomembranous candidiasis is classic form of oral candidiasis, commonly referred to as thrush. Overall, this is the most common type of oral candidiasis, accounting for about 35% of oral candidiasis cases.

It is characterized by a coating or individual patches of pseudomembranous white slough which can be easily wiped away to reveal erythematous and sometimes minimally bleeding mucosa beneath. These areas of pseudomembrane are sometimes described as "curdled milk", or "cottage cheese". The white material is made up of debris, fibrin, and desquamated epithelium which has been invaded by yeast cells and hyphae which invade to the depth of the stratum spinosum. Due to the fact that an erythematous surface is revealed beneath the pseudomembranes, some consider pseudomembranous candidiasis and erythematous candidiasis to be stages of the same entity. Some sources state that if there is bleeding when the pseudomembrane is removed, then the mucosa has likely been affected by an underlying process such as lichen planus or chemotherapy. Pseudomembraneous candidiasis can involve any part of the mouth, but usually it appears on the tongue, buccal mucosae or palate.

It is classically an acute condition, appearing in infants, people taking antibiotics or immunosuppressant medications, or immunocompromising diseases. However, sometimes it can be chronic and intermittent, even lasting for many years. Chronicity of this subtype generally occurs in immunocompromised states, (e.g.leukemia, HIV) or in persons who use corticosteroids topically or by aerosol.[4] Acute and chronic pseudomembranous candidiasis are indistinguishable in appearance.

Erythematous

Erythematous (atrophic) candidiasis is where the condition appears as a red, raw-looking lesion. Some sources consider denture-related stomatitis, angular stomatitis, median rhombiod glossitis and antiobiotic-induced stomatitis to be subtypes of erythematous candidiasis, since these lesions are commonly erythematous/atrophic. It may precede the formation of a pseudomembrane, be left when the membrane is removed, or arise de novo. Some sources state that erythematous candidiasis accounts for 60% of oral candidiasis cases. Where it is associated with inhalation steroids, erythematous candidiasis commonly appears on the palate or the dorsum of the tongue. On the tongue, there is loss of the lingual papillae (depapillation), leaving a smooth area on the tongue.

Acute erythematous candidiasis usually occurs on the dorsum of the tongue in persons taking long term corticosteroids or antibiotics, but occasionally it can occur after only a few days of using a topical antibiotic. This is usually termed "antibiotic sore mouth", "antibiotic sore tongue", or "antibiotic induced stomatitis" because it is commonly painful as well as red.

Chronic erythematous candidiasis is more usually associated with denture wearing (see denture-related stomatitis).

Hyperplastic

This variant is also sometimes termed "plaque-like candidiasis" or "nodular candidiasis". The most common appearance of hyperplastic candidiasis is a persistent white plaque which does not rub off. The lesion may be rough or nodular in texture. Hyperplastic candidiasis is uncommon, accounting for about 5% of oral candidiasis cases, and is usually chronic and found in adults. The most common site of involvement is the commisural region of the buccal mucosa, usually on both sides of the mouth.

Another term for hyperplastic candidiasis is "candidal leukoplakia". This term is a largely historical synonym for this subtype of candidiasis, rather than a true leukoplakia. Indeed, it can be clinically indistinguishable from true leukoplakia, but tissue biopsy shows candidal hyphae invading the epithelium. Some sources use this term to describe leukoplakia lesions that become colonized secondarily by Candida species, thereby distinguishing it from hyperplastic candidiasis. It is known that candida resides more readily in mucosa which is altered, such as may occur with dysplasia and hyperkeratosis in an area of leukoplakia.

Candida-associated lesions

Candida-associated lesions are primary oral candidiases (confined to the mouth), where the causes are thought to be multiple. For example, bacteria as well as candida species may be involved in these lesions. Frequently, antifungal therapy alone will not lead to permanent resolution of these lesions, but rather the underlying predisposing factors need to be addressed in addition to treating the candidiasis.

ANGULAR CHEILITIS

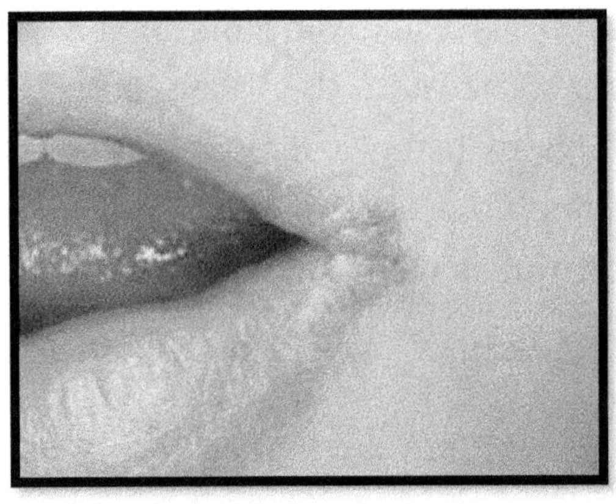

Angular cheilitis

Angular cheilitis is inflammation at the corners (angles) of the mouth, very commonly involving candida species, when sometimes the terms "candida-associated angular cheilitis", or less commonly, "monilial perlèche" are used. candida organisms alone responsible for about 20% of cases, and a mixed infection of C. albicans and Staphylococcus aureus for about 60% of cases. Signs and symptoms include soreness, erythema (redness), and fissuring of one, or more commonly both the angles of the mouth, with oedema seen intraorally on the commisures. Angular cheilitis is generally occurs in elderly people and is associated with denture related stomatitis.

Denture related stomatitis

This term refers to a mild inflammation and erythema of the mucosa beneath a denture, usually an upper denture in elderly edentulous individuals (with no natural teeth remaining). Some report that up to 65% of denture wearers have this condition to some degree. About 90% of cases are associated with candida species, where sometimes the terms "candida-associated denture stomatitis", or "Candida-associated denture induced stomatitis" (CADIS) are used. Some sources state that this is by far the most common form of oral candidiasis. Although this condition is also known as "denture sore mouth", there is rarely any pain. Candida is associated with about 90% of cases of denture related stomatitis.

Median rhomboid glossitis

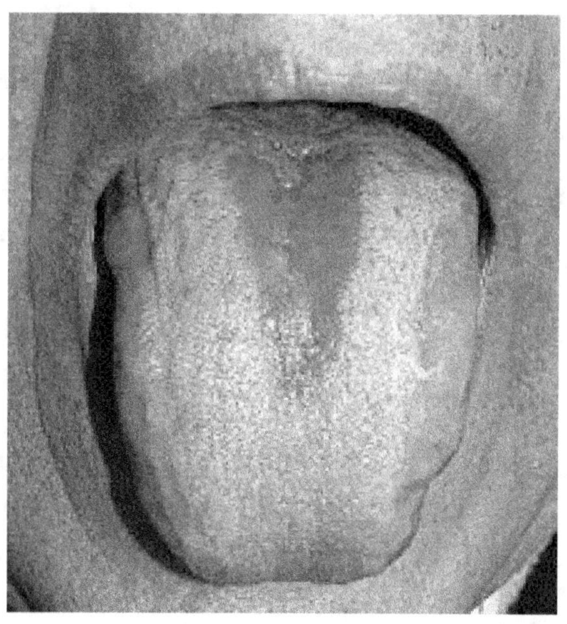

Median rhomboid glossitis

This is an elliptical or rhomboid lesion in the center of the dorsal tongue, just anterior (in front) of the circumvallate papillae. The area is depapillated, reddened (or red and white) and rarely painful. There is frequently Candida species in the lesion, sometimes mixed with bacteria.

Linear gingival erythema

This is a localized or generalized, linear band of erythematous gingivitis (inflammation of the gums). It was first observed in HIV infected individuals and termed "HIV-gingivitis", but the condition is not confined to this group. Candida species are involved, and in some cases the lesion responds to antifungal therapy, but it is thought that other factors exist, such as oral hygiene and human herpesviruses. This condition can develop into necrotizing ulcerative periodontitis.

Others

Chronic multifocal oral candidiasis

This is an uncommon form of chronic (more than one month in duration) candidial infection involving multiple areas in the mouth, without signs of candidiasis on other mucosal or cutaneous sites. The lesions are variably red and/or white. Unusually for candidal infections, there is an absence of predisposing factors such as immunosuppression, and it occurs in apparently healthy individuals, normally elderly males. Smoking is a known risk factor.

Chronic mucocutaneous candidiasis

This refers to a group of rare syndromes characterized by chronic candidal lesions on the skin, in the mouth and on other mucous membranes (i.e. a secondary oral candidiasis). These include Localized chronic mucocutaneous candidiasis, diffuse mucocutaneous candidiasis (Candida granuloma), candidiasis–endocrinopathy syndrome and candidiasis thymoma syndrome. About 90% of people with chronic mucocutaneous candidiasis will have candidiasis in the mouth.

Signs and symptoms:

Signs and symptoms are dependent upon the type of oral candidiasis. Often, apart from the appearance of the lesions, there are no other signs or symptoms. Most types of oral candidiasis are painless, but a burning sensation may occur in some cases. Candidiasis can therefore sometimes be misdiagnosed as burning mouth syndrome. A burning sensation is more likely with erythematous (atrophic) candidiasis, whilst hyperplastic candidiasis is normally entirely asymptomatic. Acute atrophic candidiasis may feel like the mouth has been scalded with a hot liquid. Another potential symptom is a metallic, acidic, salty or bitter taste in the mouth. The pseudomembranous type rarely causes any symptoms apart from possibly some discomfort or bad taste due to the presence of the membranes.[6][5] Sometimes the raised pseudomembranes will be felt by the person and described as "blisters". Occasionally there can be dysphagia (difficulty swallowing), which indicates that the candidiasis involves the oropharynx or the esophagus, as well as the mouth. The trachea ad the larynx may also be involved where there is oral candidiasis, and this may cause horseness of the voice.

Causes

Candida species: commensalism vs pathogenicity

The causative organism is usually Candida albicans, or less commonly other Candida species such as (in decreasing order of frequency): Candida tropicalis, Candida glabrata, Candida parapsilosis, Candida krusei, or other species (Candida stellatoidea, Candida pseudotropicalis, Candida famata, Candida rugosa, Candida geotrichium Candida dubliniensis, and Candida guilliermondii). C. albicans accounts for about 50% of oral candidiasis cases, and together, C. albicans, C. tropicalis and C. glabrata account for over 80% of cases. Candidiasis caused by non-C. albicans Candida (NCAC) species is associated more with immunodeficiency. For example, in HIV/AIDS, C. dubliniensis and C. geotrichium can become pathogenic.

About 35-50% of humans possess C. albicans as part of their normal oral microbiota. With more sensitive detection techniques, this figure is reported to rise to 90%. This candial carrier state is not considered to be a disease since there are no lesions or symptoms of any kind. Oral carriage of candida is pre-requisite for the development of oral candidiasis. In order for candida species to colonize and survive as a normal component of the oral microbiota, the organisms must be capable of adhering to the epithelial surface of the mucous membrane lining the mouth. This adhesion involves adhesins (e.g. hyphal wall protein 1), and extracellular polymeric materials (e.g. mannoprotein). Therefore, stains of candida which more adhesion potential are more pathogenic than other strains. The prevalence of candida carriage varies with geographic location, and many other factors. Higher carriage is reported during the summer months, in females, in hospitalized individuals, in persons with blood group O and in nonsecreterion of blood group antigens in saliva. Increased rates of candida carriage are also found in people who eat a diet high in carbohydrates, people who wear dentures, people with xerostomia (dry mouth), in people taking broad spectrum antibiotics, smokers, and in immunocompromised individuals (e.g. due to HIV/AIDS, diabetes, cancer, Down syndrome or malnutrition). Age also influences oral carriage, with the lowest levels occurring in new-borns, increasing dramatically in infants, and then decreasing again in adults. Investigations have quantified oral carriage of candida albicans at 300-500 colony forming units in healthy persons. More candida is detected in the early morning and the late afternoon. The greatest quantity of candida species is harboured on the posterior dorsal tongue, followed by the palatal and the buccal mucosae. Mucosa which is covered by an oral appliance such as a denture harbours significantly more candida species than uncovered mucosa.

When candida species cause lesions- the result of invasion of the host tissues- this is termed candidiasis. Some consider oral candidiasis to be a change in the normal oral environment rather than an exposure or true "infection" as such. The exact process by which Candida species switch from acting as a normal oral commensal in the carrier (saprophytic) state to acting as a pathogenic organism (parasitic state) is not completely understood.

Several candida species are polymorphogenic, that is, capable of growing in different forms depending on the environmental conditions. C. albicans can appear as a yeast form (blastospores), which is thought to be relatively harmless; and a hyphal form which is associated with invasion of host tissues. Apart from true hyphae, Candida can also form pseudohyphae which are elongated filamentous cells, lined end to end. As a general rule, candidiasis presenting with white lesions is mainly caused by Candida species in the hyphal form and red lesions by yeast forms. C. albicans and C. dubliniensis are also capable of forming germ tubes (incipient hyphae) and chlamydospores under the right conditions. Pseudohyphae are elongated filamentous cells, lined end to end. C. albicans is categorized serologically into A and B serotypes. The prevalence is roughly equal in healthy individuals, but type B is more prevalent in immunocompromised individuals.

Predisposing factors

Common local and systemic predisposing factors	
Local host factors - Dentures - Corticosteroid inhalers - Reduced salivary flow - High sugar diet	Systemic host factors - Extremes of age - Endocrine disorders (e.g. diabetes) - Immunosuppression - Broad spectrum antibiotics (e.g. tetracycline) Nutritional deficiencies

The host defences against opportunistic infection of candida species are comprised of:

- The oral epithelium, which acts both as a physical barrier preventing micro-organisms from entering the tissues, and is the site of cell mediated immune reactions.
- Competition and inhibition interactions between candida species and other micro-organisms in the mouth, such as the many hundreds of different kinds of bacteria.
- Saliva, which possesses both mechanical cleansing action and immunologic action, including salivary immunoglobulin A antibodies, which aggregate candida organisms and prevent them adhering to the epithelial surface; and enzymatic components such as lysozyme, lactoperoxidase and antileukoprotease. Disruption to any of these local and systemic host defence mechanisms constitutes a potential susceptibility to oral candidiasis, which rarely occurs without predisposing factors. It is often described as being "a disease of the diseased", occurring in the very young, the very old, or the very sick.

Immunodeficiency / immunocompromise

Acute pseudomembranous candidiasis occurs in about 5% of new-born infants. Candida species are acquired from the mother's vaginal canal during birth. At very young ages, the immune system is yet to develop fully and there is no "immunity" to candida species.

Immunocompromise, e.g. as a result of AIDS/HIV or chemotherapy.

Topical or systemic corticosteroids, e.g. for treatment of asthma or COPD may also result in oral candidiasis: the risk may be reduced by regularly rinsing the mouth with water after taking the medication.

Active cancer and treatment, chemotherapy or radiotherapy.

Denture wearing

Denture wearing, and poor denture hygiene, particularly wearing the denture continually rather than removing them during sleep, is another risk factor, both for candidal carriage and for oral candidiasis. Dentures provide a relative acidic, moist and anaerobic environment because the mucosa covered by the denture is sheltered from oxygen and saliva. Loose, poorly fitting dentures may also cause minor trauma to the mucosa, which is thought to increase the permeability of the mucosa and increase the ability of C. albicans to invade the tissues. These conditions all favour the growth of C. albicans. Sometimes dentures become very worn, or they have been constructed to allow insufficient lower facial height (occlusal vertical dimension), leading to over-closure of the mouth (an appearance sometimes described as "collapse of the jaws"). This causes pronouncement of the skin folds at the corners of the mouth, in effect creating an intertriginous areas in which another form of candidiasis, angular cheilitis, can develop. Candida species are capable of adhering to the surface of dentures, most of which are made from polymethyl acrylate. They exploit micro-fissures and cracks in the surface of dentures to aid their retention. Intra-oral prostheses may therefore become covered in a biofilm, and act as reservoirs of infection, continually re-infecting the mucosa. For this reason, disinfecting the denture is a vital part of treatment of oral candidiasis in persons who wear dentures, as well as correcting other factors like inadequate lower facial height and fit of the dentures.

DRY MOUTH

Both the quantity and quality of saliva are important oral defences against candida. Decreased salivary flow rate or a change in the composition of saliva, collectively termed salivary hypofunction or hyposalivation is an important predisposing factor. Xerostomia is frequently listed as a cause of candidiasis, but xerostomia can be subjective or objective, i.e. a symptom presents with or without actual changes in the saliva consistency or flow rate.

Diet

Malnutrition, whether by malabsorption, or poor diet, especially hematinic deficiencies (iron, vitamin B12, folic acid) can predispose to oral candidiasis, by causing diminished host defence and epithelial integrity. For example, iron deficiency anaemia is thought to cause depressed cell-mediated immunity. Some sources state that deficiencies of vitamin A or pyroxidine are also linked.

There is limited evidence that a diet high in carbohydrates predisposes to oral candidiasis. In vitro and studies show that Candidal growth, adhesion and biofilm formation is enhanced by the presence of carbohydrates such as glucose, galactose and sucrose.

Smoking

Smoking, especially heavy smoking, is an important predisposing factor but the reasons for this relationship are unknown. One hypothesis is that cigarette smoke contains nutritional factors for C. albicans, or that local epithelial alterations occur which facilitate colonization of candida species.

Antibiotics

Imbalance of the oral microbiota. Broad-spectrum antibiotics which eliminate the competing bacteria and disrupt the normally balanced ecology of oral micro-organisms. acute oral candidiasis occurring due to medication with corticosteroids or broad-spectrum antibiotics (e.g. tetracycline). There is generalized mucosal erythema and soreness, sometimes with areas of pseudomembranous candidiasis. Antibiotic or steroid-induced stomatitis

Other factors

Endocrine disorders, e.g. diabetes (when poorly controlled).

Presence of certain other mucosal lesions, especially those which cause hyperkeratosis and/or dysplasia, e.g. lichen planus. Such changes in the mucosa predispose it to secondary infection with candidiasis. Other physical mucosal alterations are sometimes associated with candida overgrowth, such as Fissured tongue (rarely), or Tongue piercing.

Women undergoing hormonal changes, like pregnancy or those on birth control pills Atopy. Hospitalization. Lupus.

Diagnosis

The diagnosis can typically be made from the clinical appearance alone, but not always. As candidiasis can be variable in appearance, and present with white, red or combined white and red lesions, the differential diagnosis can be extensive. In pseudomembranous candidiasis, the membranous slough can be wiped away to reveal an erythematous surface underneath. This is helpful in distinguishing pseudomembranous candidiasis from other white lesions in the mouth that cannot be wiped away, such as lichen planus, oral hairy leukoplakia. Erythematous candidiasis can mimic geographic tongue. Erythematous candidiasis usually has a diffuse border, helping to distinguish it from erythroplakia which normally has a sharply defined border.

Special investigations to detect the presence of candida species include oral swabs, oral rinse or oral smears. Smears are collected by gentle scraping of the lesion with a spatula or tongue blade and the resulting debris directly applied to a glass slide. Oral swabs are taken if culture is required. Some recommend that swabs be taken from 3 different oral sites. Oral rinse involves rinsing the mouth with phosphate-buffered saline for 1 minute and then spitting out the solution again into a vessel which is sent to the pathology laboratory for examination. Oral rinse technique is capable of distinguishing between commensal candidal carriage and candidiasis. If candidal leukoplakia is suspected, a biopsy may be indicated. Smears and biopsies are usually stained with Periodic acid-Schiff which stains cabohydrate in fungal cell walls magenta. Gram staining is also used as Candida stains strongly Gram +ve. Sometimes an underlying medical condition is sought, and this may include blood tests for full blood count and hematinics.

If a biopsy is taken, the histopathologic appearance can be variable depending upon the clinical type of candidiasis. Pseudomembranous candidiasis shows hyperplastic epithelium with a superficial parakeratotic desquamating (i.e. separating) layer. Hyphae penetrate to the depth of the stratum spinosum, and appear as weakly basophilic structures. Polymorphonuclear cells also infiltrate the epithelium, and chronic inflammatory cells infiltrate the lamina propria.

Atrophic candidiasis appears as thin, atrophic epithelium which is non keratinized. Hyphae are sparse, and inflammatory cell infiltration of the epithelium and the lamina propria. In essence, atrophic candidiasis appears like pseudomembranous candidiasis without the superficial desquamating layer.

Hyperplastic candidiasis is variable. Usually there is hyperplastic and acanthotic epithelium with parakeratosis. There is an inflammatory cell infiltrate and hypae are visible. Unlike other forms of candidiasis, hyperplastic candidiasis may show dysplasia.

Treatment

Oral candidiasis can be treated with topical anti-fungal drugs, such as nystatin, miconazole, Gentian violet or amphotericin B.

Patients who are immunocompromised, either with HIV/AIDS or as a result of chemotherapy, may require systemic treatment with oral or intravenous administered anti-fungals.

If candidiasis is secondary to corticosteroid or antibiotic use, this may be stopped, although often this is not a feasible option depending on the initial reason the drug was prescribed. Underlying immunosuppression may be medically manageable once it is identified, and this will help to prevent recurrence of candidal infections.

In recurrent oral candidiasis, the use of azole antifungals risks selection and enrichment of drug-resistant strains of candida organisms. Drug resistance is increasingly more common and presents a serious problem in persons who are immunocompromised.

Prophylactic use of antifungals is sometimes employed in persons with HIV disease, during radiotherapy, during immunosuppressive or prolonged antibiotic therapy as the development of candidal infection in these groups may be more serious.

The Candida load in the mouth can be reduced by improving oral hygiene measures, such as regular toothbrushing and use of anti-microbial mouthwashes. Since smoking is associated with many of forms of oral candidiasis, cessation may be beneficial. In individuals who have developed candidiasis secondary to the use of inhaled steroids, rinsing out the mouth with water after taking the steroid, and using a spacer device to reduce the contact with the oral mucosa (particularly the dorsal tongue) may be beneficial.

Denture hygiene

Good denture hygiene involves regular cleaning of the dentures, and leaving them out of the mouth during sleep. This gives the mucosa a chance to recover, whilst wearing a denture during sleep is often likened to sleeping in one's shoes. In oral candidiasis, the dentures may act as a reservoir of Candida species, continually reinfecting the mucosa once antifungal medication is stopped. Therefore, they need to be disinfected as part of the treatment for oral candidiasis. There are commercial preparations for this purpose, but it is readily accomplished by soaking the denture overnight in a 1:10 solution of sodium hypochlorite (Milton, or household bleach). Bleach may corrode metal components, so if the denture contains metal, soaking it twice daily inchlorhexidine solution can be carried out instead. An alternative method of disinfection is to use a 10% solution of acetic acid (vinegar) as an overnight soak, or to microwave the dentures in 200mL water for 3 minutes at 650 watts. Antifungal medication can also be applied to the fitting surface of the denture before it is put back in the mouth. Other problems with the dentures, such as inadequate occlusal vertical dimension may also need to be corrected in the case of angular cheilitis.

Prognosis

The severity of oral candidiasis is subject to great variability, from one person to another, and in the same person from one occasion to the next. The prognosis of such infection is usually excellent after the application of topical or systemic treatments. However, oral candidiasis can be recurrent. Individuals will continue to at risk of the condition if the underlying factors such as reduced salivary flow rate or immunosuppression are not rectifiable.

Candidiasis can be a marker for underlying disease, so the overall prognosis may also be dependent upon this. For example, a transient erythematous candidiasis which developed after antiobiotic therapy will usually resolve after the antibiotics are stopped (but not always immediately), and therefore carries an excellent prognosis, but candidiasis may occasionally be a herald of a more sinister undiagnosed pathology such as HIV/AIDS or leukemia.

It is possible for candidiasis to spread to/from the mouth, from sites such as the pharynx, esophagus, lungs, liver, anogenital region, skin or the nails. The spread of oral candidiasis to other sites is usually occurs in debilitated individuals. It is also possible that candidiasis is spread by sexual contact. Rarely, a superficial candidal infection such as oral candidiasis can cause invasive, and even prove fatal. The observation that Candida species are normally harmless commensals on the one hand, but are also occasionally capable of causing fatal invasive candidiasis.

The role of thrush in the hospital and ventilated patients is not entirely clear however there is a theoretical risk of positive interaction of candida with topical bacteria that could increase the risk for Ventilator Associated Pneumonia and other diseases.

GINGIVITIS

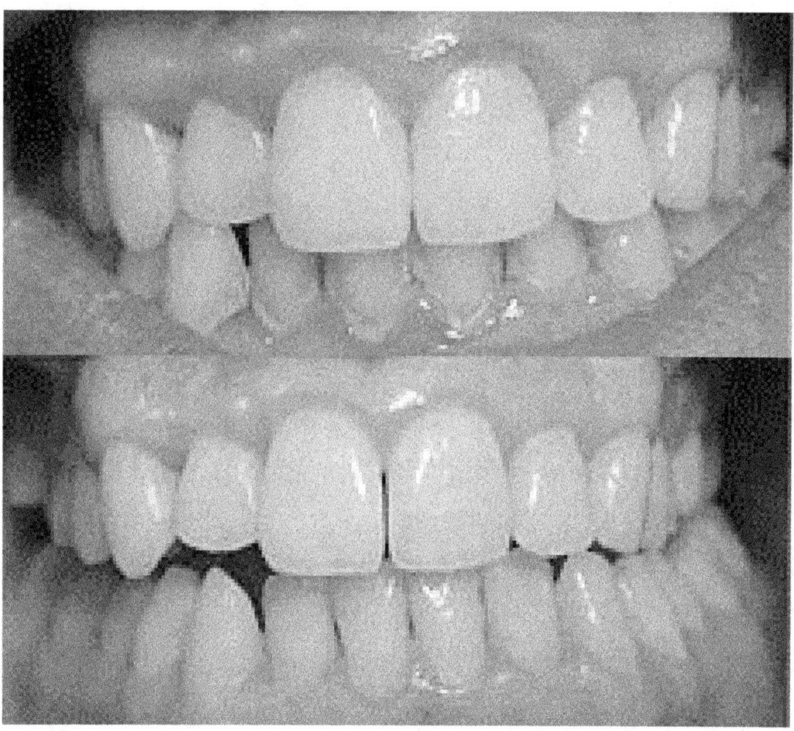

Gingivitis ("inflammation of the gum tissue") is a non-destructive periodontal disease. The most common form of gingivitis, and the most common form of periodontal disease overall, is in response to bacterial biofilms (also called plaque) adherent to tooth surfaces, termed plaque-induced gingivitis. In the absence of treatment, gingivitis may progress to periodontitis, which is a destructive form of periodontal disease.

While in some sites or individuals' gingivitis never progresses to periodontitis, data indicates that periodontitis is always preceded by gingivitis

As defined by the 1999 World Workshop in Clinical Periodontics, there are two primary categories of gingival diseases, each with numerous subgroups:

Classification

1. **Dental plaque-induced gingival diseases**
   - Gingivitis associated with plaque only
   - Gingival diseases modified by systemic factors
   - Gingival diseases modified by medications
   - Gingival diseases modified by malnutrition
2. **Non-plaque-induced gingival lesions**
   - Gingival diseases of specific bacterial origin
   - Gingival diseases of viral origin
   - Gingival diseases of fungal origin
   - Gingival diseases of genetic origin
   - Gingival manifestations of systemic conditions
   - Traumatic lesions
   - Foreign body reactions
   - Not otherwise specified

Signs and symptoms

The symptoms of gingivitis are somewhat non-specific and manifest in the gum tissue as the classic signs of inflammation:

- Swollen gums
- Bright red or purple gums
- Gums that are tender or painful to the touch
- Bleeding gums or bleeding after brushing and/or flossing
- Bad breath (halitosis)

Additionally, the stippling that normally exists on the gum tissue of some individuals will often disappear and the gums may appear shiny when the gum tissue becomes swollen and stretched over the inflamed underlying connective tissue. The accumulation may also emit an unpleasant odour. When the gingiva are swollen, the epithelial lining of the gingival crevice becomes ulcerated and the gums will bleed more easily with even gentle brushing, and especially when flossing.

Causes

The etiology, or cause, of plaque-induced gingivitis is bacterial plaque, which acts to initiate the body's host response. This, in turn, can lead to destruction of the gingival tissues, which may progress to destruction of the periodontal attachment apparatus. The plaque accumulates in the small gaps between teeth, in the gingival grooves and in areas known as plaque traps: locations that serve to accumulate and maintain plaque. Examples of plaque traps include bulky and overhanging restorative margins, claps of removable partial dentures and calculus (tartar) that forms on teeth. Although these accumulations may be tiny, the bacteria in them produce chemicals, such as degrative enzymes, and toxins, such as lipopolysaccharide (LPS, otherwise known asendotoxin) or lipoteichoic acid (LTA), that promote an inflammatory response in the gum tissue. This inflammation can cause an enlargement of the gingiva and subsequent formation.

Diagnosis

A dental hygienist or dentist will check for the symptoms of gingivitis, and may also examine the amount of plaque in the oral cavity. A dental hygienist or dentist will also look for signs of periodontitis using X-rays or periodontal probing as well as other methods.

If gingivitis is not responsive to treatment, referral to a periodontist (a specialist in diseases of the gingiva and bone around teeth and dental implants) for further treatment may be necessary.

Prevention

Gingivitis can be prevented through regular oral hygiene that includes daily brushing and flossing. Hydrogenperoxide, saline, alcohol or chlorhexidine m outh washes may also be employed. In a recent clinical study, the beneficial effect of hydrogen peroxide on gingivitis has been highlighted. Rigorous plaque control programs along with periodontal scaling and curettage also have proved to be helpful, although according to the American Dental Association, periodontal scaling and root planning are considered as a treatment to periodontal disease, not as a preventive treatment for periodontal disease. In a 1997 review of effectiveness data the U.S. Food and Drug Administration (FDA) found clear evidence which showed that toothpaste containing triclosan was effective in preventing gingivitis.

In many countries, such as the United States, mouthwashes containing chlorhexidine are available only by prescription.

Researchers analysed government data on calcium consumption and periodontal disease indicators in nearly 13,000 U.S. adults. They found that men and women who had calcium intakes of fewer than 500 milligrams, or about half the recommended dietary allowance, were almost twice as likely to have gum disease, as measured by the loss of attachment of the gums from the teeth. The association was particularly evident for people in their 20s and 30s.

Preventing gum disease may also benefit a healthy heart. According to physicians with The Institute for Good Medicine at the Pennsylvania Medical Society, good oral health can reduce risk of cardiac events. Poor oral health can lead to infections that can travel within the bloodstream.

Treatment

Analgesic and antiseptic gum paint with applicator buds used in treatment of gingivitis. The focus of treatment for gingivitis is removal of the etiologic (causative) agent, plaque. Therapy is aimed at the reduction of oral bacteria, and may take the form of regular periodic visits to a dental professional together with adequate oral hygiene home care. Thus, several of the methods used in the prevention of gingivitis can also be used for the treatment of manifest gingivitis, such as scaling, root planning, curettage, mouth washes containing chlorhexidine or hydrogen peroxide, and flossing. Interdental brushes also help remove any causative agents.

Recent scientific studies have also shown the beneficial effects of mouthwashes with essential oils.

Furthermore, oral Non-Steroidal Anti-Inflammatory Drug (NSAID) rinses are a relatively new treatment modality for treating inflammation in the oral cavity. NSAIDs such as ibuprofen or diclofenac, are a mainstay of analgesic and anti-inflammatory treatment in dentistry. However, the systemic use of NSAID's are associated with several side-effects, namely cardiovascular thrombotic events, such as myocardial infarction and stroke, gastric irritability or ulcerogenic effects, blood dyscrasias, and nephrotoxicity; among these gastric irritability is most common. Therefore, it is preferable to use local formulations such as a mouthwash to treat oral inflammatory conditions e.g. gingivitis. A randomized, investigator-blind, clinical study published in September, 2011, showed the new Diclofenac Epolamine (diclofenac N-(2-hydroxyethyl) Pyrrolidine; DHEP), a diclofenac salt with greater water solubility, as an effective and tolerable medicinal product for symptomatic and post-surgical relief of inflammation of the oral cavity. Volunteers with inflammatory conditions, of which gingivitis was most prevalent, treated with DHEP, experienced a significantly greater reduction in pain and inflammation and were also free of pain and inflammatory symptoms as soon as Day 3 of the study compared to those treated with merely 0.0075% diclofenac mouthwash. There was an even greater reduction relative to the placebo group.

Complications

o Tooth loss, or decay
o Recurrence of gingivitis
o Periodontitis
o Infection or abscess of the gingiva or the jaw bones
o Trench mouth (bacterial infection and ulceration of the gums)
o swollen glands

GLOSSITIS

Glossitis is a condition in which the tongue is swollen and changes colour, often making the surface of the tongue appear smooth.

Alternative Names

Tongue inflammation, Tongue infection, Smooth tongue, Glossodynia, Burning tongue syndrome

Causes

Glossitis is often a symptom of other conditions or problems, including:

- Allergic reaction to toothpaste, mouthwash, breath fresheners, dyes in candy, plastic in dentures or retainers, or certain blood pressure medications (ACE inhibitors)
- Dry mouth, when the glands that produce saliva are destroyed
- Infections with bacteria or viruses (including oral herpes simplex)
- Injury from burns, rough edges of teeth or dental appliances, or other trauma
- Low iron levels (called iron deficiency) or certain B vitamins, such as vitamin B12
- Skin conditions such as oral lichen planus, erythema multiform, aphthous ulcers, pemphigus vulgaris, syphilis, and others
- Tobacco, alcohol, hot foods, spices, or other irritants
- Yeast infection in the mouth

At times, glossitis may be passed down in families and is not due to another disease or event.

Symptoms

Symptoms of glossitis may appear quickly or slowly over time. They include:

- Difficulty with chewing, swallowing, or speaking
- Smooth surface of the tongue
- Sore and tender tongue
- Tongue colour changes
    - Pale, if caused by pernicious anaemia
    - Fiery red, if caused by a lack of other B vitamins
- Tongue swelling

Exams and Tests

An examination by a dentist or health care provider shows:

- Finger-like bumps on the surface of the tongue (called papillae) may be missing
- Swollen tongue (or patches of swelling)

Your health care provider may ask detailed questions about your medical history and lifestyle to find the cause of tongue inflammation if there was no obvious injury or other cause.

Blood tests may be done to rule out other medical conditions.

Treatment

The goal of treatment is to reduce inflammation. Most people do not need to go to the hospital for treatment unless tongue swelling is severe.

- Good oral hygiene is important. Brush your teeth thoroughly at least twice a day and floss at least once a day.
- Antibiotics, antifungal medications, or other antimicrobials may be prescribed if the glossitis is due to an infection.
- Dietary changes and supplements are used to treat anaemia and nutritional deficiencies.
- Avoid irritants (such as hot or spicy foods, alcohol, and tobacco) to reduce any tongue discomfort.

Outlook (Prognosis)

Glossitis usually responds well to treatment if the cause of inflammation is removed or treated. This disorder may be painless, or it may cause tongue and mouth discomfort. In some cases, glossitis may result in severe tongue swelling that blocks the airway.

Possible Complications
- Airway blockage
- Difficulties with speaking, chewing, or swallowing
- Discomfort

Prevention

Good oral hygiene (thorough tooth brushing and flossing and regular professional cleaning and examination) may help prevent glossitis.

LEUKOPLAKIA

Leukoplakia are patches on the tongue, in the mouth, or on the inside of the cheek that occur in response to long-term irritation. Leukoplakia patches may also develop on the outer female genitals.

Alternative Names

Hairy leucoplakia, Smoker's keratosis, Vulvar leukoplakia

Causes

Leukoplakia mainly affects the mucus membranes of the mouth. It is thought to be caused by irritation, but the cause is not always known.

Irritation in the mouth may be caused by:

- Rough teeth
- Rough places on dentures, fillings, and crowns
- Smoking or other tobacco use (smoker's keratosis), especially pipes
- Holding chewing tobacco or snuff in your mouth for a long period of time

The disorder is most common in elderly persons.

"Hairy" leukoplakia of the mouth is a different disorder that is seen mostly in HIV-positive people. It may be one of the first signs of HIV infection. It can also appear in other people whose immune system is not working well, such as after a bone marrow transplant. It is caused by the Epstein-Barr virus, but is not harmful by itself. The most common symptoms of hairy leukoplakia are painless, fuzzy white patches on the side of the tongue.

Symptoms

Sores usually develop on the tongue, but they may also appear on the insides of the cheek, or on the outer female genitals. The most common symptoms of hairy leukoplakia are painless, fuzzy white patches on the side of the tongue.

The sores are,

- Usually white or grey
- Sometimes red (called erythroplakia, a condition that can lead to cancer)
- Thick and slightly raised with a hard surface that can't be easily scraped off

Exams and Tests

The typical white patch of leukoplakia develops slowly, over weeks to months. The lesion may eventually become rough in texture, and may become sensitive to touch, heat, spicy foods, or other irritation.

A biopsy of the lesion confirms the diagnosis. An examination of the biopsy specimen may find changes that indicate oral cancer.

Treatment

The goal of treatment is to get rid of the lesion. Removing the source of irritation is important and may cause the lesion to disappear.

- Treat dental causes such as rough teeth, irregular denture surface, or fillings as soon as possible.
- Stop smoking or using other tobacco products.
- Do not drink alcohol.

Outlook (Prognosis)

Leukoplakia is usually harmless. Lesions often clear up in a few weeks or months after the source of irritation is removed. Rarely, it may become cancer.

Prevention

Stop smoking or using other tobacco products. Do not drink alcohol, or limit your number of alcoholic drinks. Have rough teeth treated and dental appliances repaired promptly.

MOUTH ULCERS

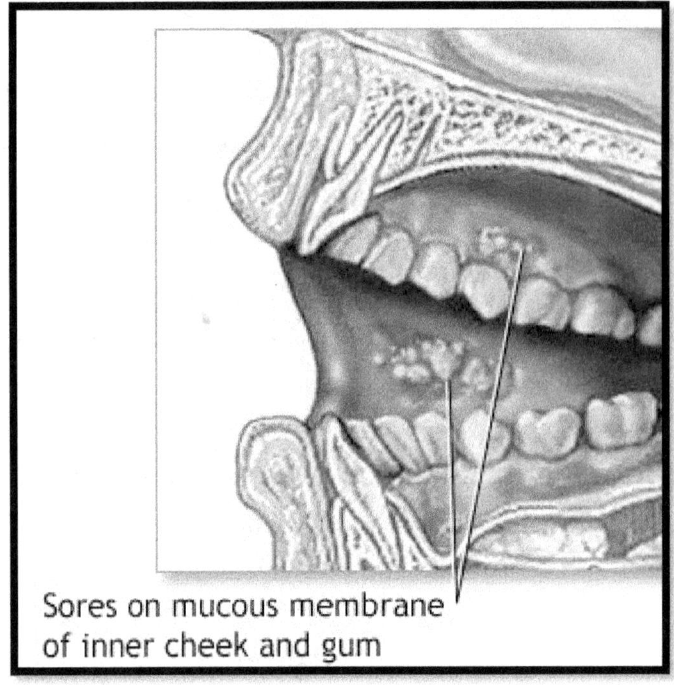

Causes

Mouth ulcers are caused by many disorders. These include:

- Canker sores
- Gingivostomatitis
- Herpes simplex (fever blister)
- Leukoplakia
- Oral cancer
- Oral lichen planus
- Oral thrush

The skin lesion of histoplasmosis may also appear as a mouth ulcer.

Symptoms

Symptoms vary and depend on the specific cause of the mouth ulcer. In general, symptoms may include:
- Open sores in the mouth
- Pain or discomfort in the mouth

Exams and Tests

A health care provider or dentist usually diagnoses the type of mouth ulcer, based on its appearance and location. Blood tests or a biopsy of the ulcer may be needed to confirm the cause.

Treatment

The goal of treatment is to relieve symptoms. The cause, if known, should be treated.

Gentle, thorough oral hygiene may relieve some of the symptoms. Topical (rubbed on) antihistamines, antacids, corticosteroids, or other soothing preparations may be recommended for applying directly to the ulcer.

Avoid hot or spicy foods, which often increase the pain of mouth ulcers.

Prognosis

The outcome varies depending on the cause of the ulcer. Many mouth ulcers are harmless and heal without treatment.

There are types of cancer, however, that may first appear as a mouth ulcer that does not heal. See: Squamous cell carcinoma

Possible Complications

- Cellulitis of the mouth, from secondary bacterial infection of ulcers
- Dental infections (tooth abscesses)
- Oral cancer
- Spread of contagious disorders to other people

Prevention

Good oral hygiene may help prevent some types of mouth ulcers, as well as some complications from mouth ulcers. Good oral hygiene includes brushing the teeth at least twice per day, flossing at least daily, and getting regular professional dental cleanings and examinations.

SIALOLITHIASIS

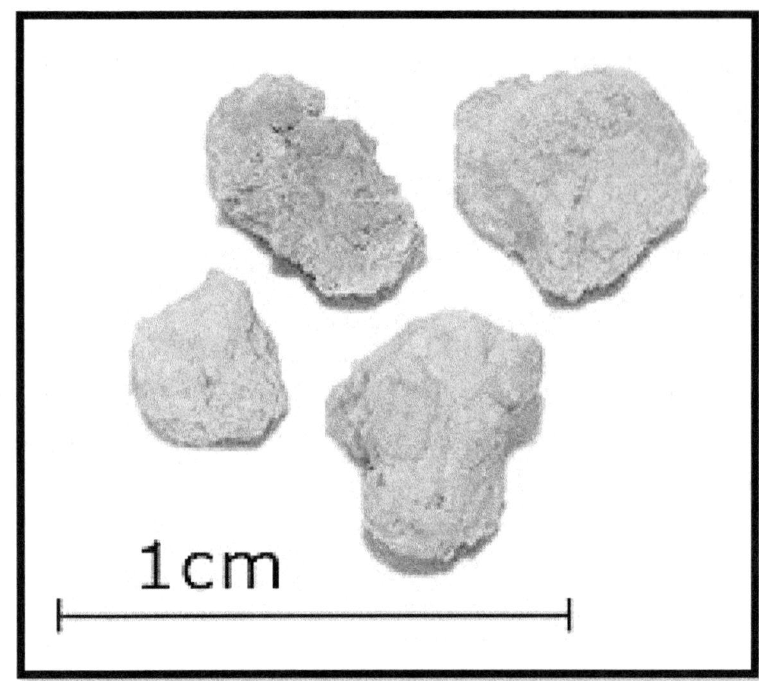

Calculi (salivary gland stones) removed from the sublingual gland

Sialolithiasis (also termed **salivary calculi**, or **salivary stones**), is a condition where a calcified mass forms within a salivary gland, usually in the duct of the submandibular gland (also termed "Wharton's duct"). Less commonly the parotid gland or rarely the sublingual gland or a minor salivary gland may develop salivary stones.

The usual symptoms are pain and swelling of the affected salivary gland, both of which get worse when salivary flow is stimulated, e.g. with the sight, thought, smell or taste of food, or with hunger or chewing. This is often termed "mealtime syndrome". Inflammation or infection of the gland may develop as a result. Sialolithiasis may also develop because of the presence of existing chronic infection of the glands, dehydration (e.g. use of phenothiazines), Sjögren's syndrome and/or increased local levels of calcium, but in many instances the cause is idiopathic (unknown).

The condition is usually managed by removing the stone, and several different techniques are available. Rarely, removal of the submandibular gland may become necessary in cases of recurrent stone formation. Sialolithiasis is common, accounting for about 50% of all disease occurring in the major salivary glands and causing symptoms in about 0.45% of the general population. Persons aged 30-60 and males are more likely to develop sialolithiasis.

The term is derived from the Greek words sialon (saliva) and lithos (stone), and the Latin -iasis meaning "process" or "morbid condition". A calculus (plural calculi) is a hard, stone-like concretionthat forms within an organ or duct inside the body. They are usually made from mineral salts, and other types of calculi include tonsiloliths (tonsil stones) and renal calculi (kidney stones). Sialolithiasis refers to the formation of calculi within a salivary gland. If a calculus forms in the duct that drains the saliva from a salivary gland into the mouth, then saliva will be trapped in the gland. This may cause painful swelling and inflammation of the gland. Inflammation of a salivary gland is termed sialadenitis. Inflammation associated with blockage of the duct is sometimes termed "obstructive sialadenitis". Because saliva is stimulated to flow more with the thought, site or smell of food, or with chewing, pain and swelling will often get suddenly worse just before and during a meal ("peri-prandial"), and then slowly decrease after eating, this is termed meal time syndrome. However, calculi are not the only reasons that a salivary gland may become blocked and give rise to the meal time syndrome. Obstructive salivary gland disease, or obstructive sialadenitis, may also occur due to fibromucinous plugs, duct stenosis, foreign bodies, anatomic variations, or malformations of the duct system leading to a mechanical obstruction associated with stasis of saliva in the duct.

Salivary stones may be divided according to which gland they form in. About 85% of stones occur in the submandibular gland and between 5-10% occur in the parotid gland. In about 0-5% of cases, the sublingual gland or a minor salivary gland is affected. When minor glands are rarely involved, caliculi are more likely in the minor glands of the buccal mucosa and the maxillary labial mucosa. Submandibular stones are further classified as anterior or posterior in relation to an imaginary transverse line drawn between the mandibular first molar teeth. Stones may beradiopaque, i.e. they will show up on conventional radiographs, or radiolucent, where they not be visible on radiographs (although some of their effects on the gland may still be visible). They may also symptomatic or asymptomatic, according to whether they cause any problems or not.

Signs and symptoms

Signs and symptoms are variable and depend largely upon whether the obstruction of the duct is complete or partial, and how much resultant pressure is created within the gland. The development of infection in the gland also influences the signs and symptoms.

- Pain, which is intermittent, and may suddenly get worse before mealtimes, and then slowly get better (partial obstruction).
- Swelling of the gland, also usually intermittent, often suddenly appearing or increasing before mealtimes, and then slowly going down (partial obstruction).
- Tenderness of the involved gland.
- Palpable hard lump, if the stone is located near the end of the duct. If the stone is near the submandibular duct orifice, the lump may be felt under the tongue.
- Lack of saliva coming from the duct (total obstruction).
- Erythema (redness) of the floor of the mouth (infection).
- Pus discharging from the duct (infection).
- Cervical lymphadenitis (infection).

Rarely, when stones form in the minor salivary glands, there is usually only slight local swelling in the form of a small nodule and tenderness.

Causes

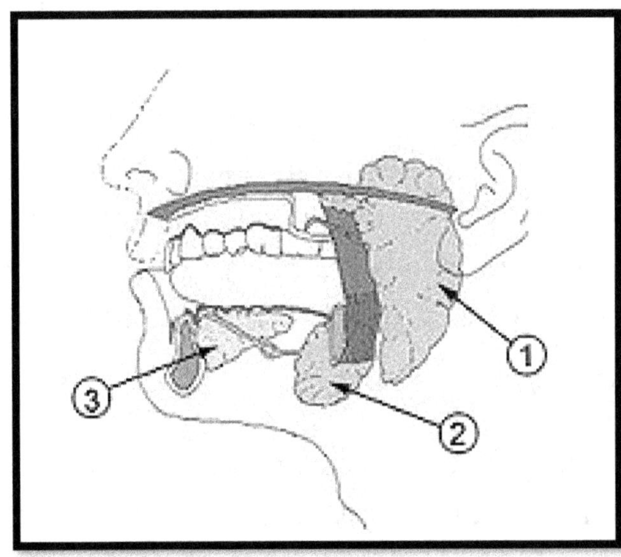

The major salivary glands (paired on each side). 1. Parotid gland, 2. Submandibular gland, 3. Sublingual gland.

There are thought to be a series of stages that lead to the formation of a calculi (lithogenesis). Initially, factors such as abnormalities in calcium metabolism, dehydration, reduced salivary flow rate, altered acidity (pH) of saliva caused by oropharyngeal infections, and altered solubility of crystalloids, leading to precipitation of mineral salts, are involved. Other sources state that no systemic abnormality of calcium or phosphate metabolism is responsible.

The next stage involves the formation of a nidus which is successively layered with organic and inorganic material, eventually forming a calcified mass. In about 15-20% of cases the sialolith will not be sufficiently calcified to appear radiopaque on a radiograph, and therefore be difficult to detect.

Other sources suggest a retrograde theory of lithogenesis, where food debris, bacteria or foreign bodies from the mouth enter the ducts of a salivary gland and are trapped by abnormalities in the sphincter mechanism of the duct opening (the papilla), which are reported in 90% of cases. Fragments of bacteria from salivary calculi were reported to be Streptococci species which are part of the normal oral microbiota and are present in dental plaque.

Stone formation occurs most commonly in the submandibular gland for several reasons. The concentration of calcium in saliva produced by the submandibular gland is twice that of the saliva produced by the parotid gland. The sumbandibular gland saliva is also relatively alkaline and mucous. The submandibular duct (Warton's duct) is long, meaning that saliva secretions must travel further before being discharged into the mouth. The duct possesses two bends, the first at the posterior border of the mylohyoid muscle and the second near the duct orifice. The flow of saliva from the submandibular gland is often against gravity due to variations in the location of the duct orifice. The orifice itself is smaller than that of the parotid.

These factors all promote slowing and stasis of saliva in the submandibular duct, making the formation of an obstruction with subsequent calcification more likely.

Salivary calculi sometimes are associated with other salivary diseases, e.g. sialoliths occur in two thirds of cases of chronic sialadenitis, although obstructive sialadenitis is often a consequence of sialolithiasis. Gout may also cause salivary stones, although in this case they are composed of uric acid crystals rather than the normal composition of salivary stones.

Diagnosis

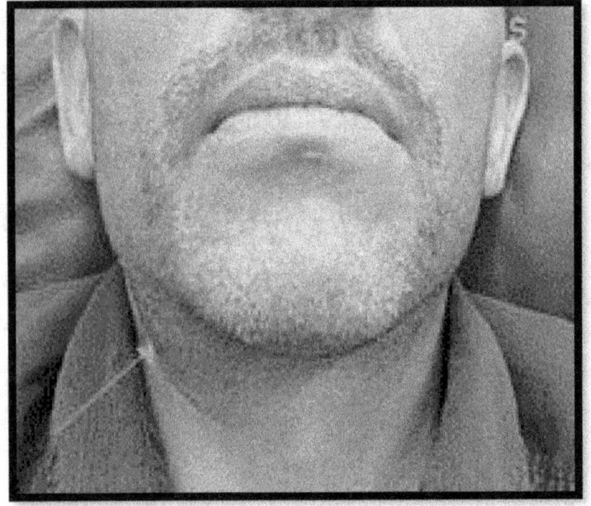

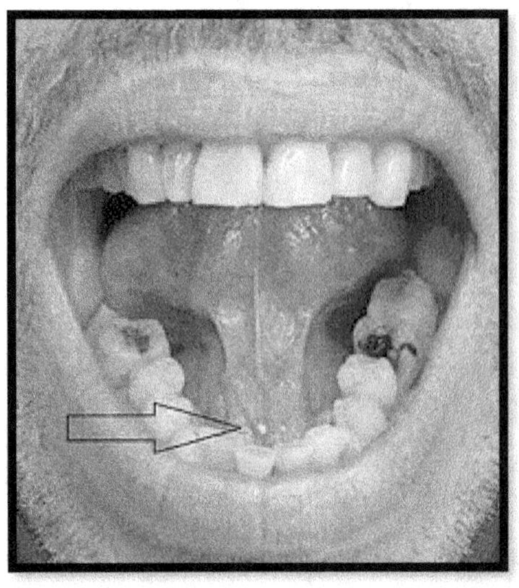

Swelling of the submandibular gland as seen from the outside

The stone seen in the submandicular duct on the right side

Diagnosis is usually made by characteristic history and physical examination. Diagnosis can be confirmed by x-ray (80% of salivary gland calculi are visible on x-ray), or by sialogram or ultrasound.

Treatment

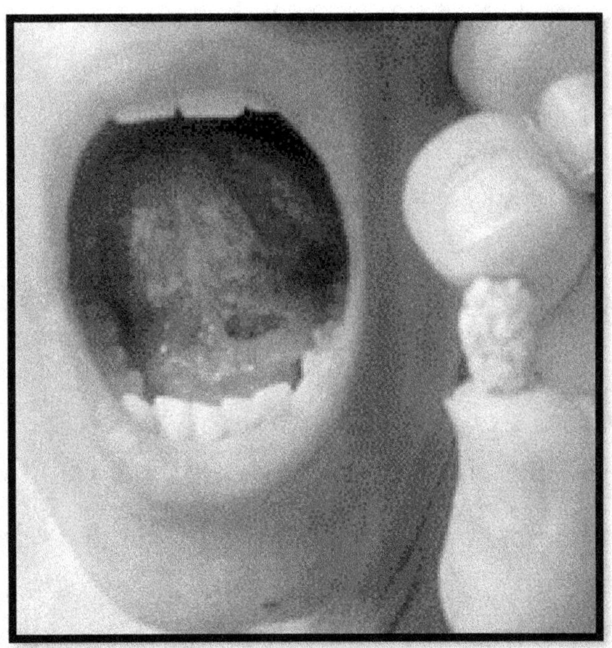

Salivary gland stone and the hole left behind from the operation

Current treatment options are:

- For small stones, hydration, moist heat, NSAIDs occasionally, and having the patient take any food or beverage that is bitter and/or sour. Sucking on citrus fruits, such as a lemon or orange, may increase salivation and promote spontaneous expulsion of the stone.
- Some stones may be massaged out by a specialist.
- An ENT or maxillofacial surgeon may canulate the duct to remove the stone (sialotomy).
- A surgeon may make a small incision near the stone to remove it.
- Sialendoscopy
- To prevent infection while the stone is lodged in the duct, sometimes antibiotics are used. In some cases when stones continually reoccur the offending salivary duct is removed.
- Shock wave therapy for disintegration of the salivary stones can also be effectively used.

Epidemiology

The prevalence of salivary stones in the general population is about 1.2% according to post mortem studies, but the prevalence of salivary stones which cause symptoms is about 0.45% in the general population. Sialolithiasis accounts for about 50% of all disease occurring in major salivary glands, and for about 66% of all obstructive salivary gland diseases. Salivary gland stones are twice as common in males as in females. The most common age range in which they occur is between 30 and 60, and they are uncommon in children.

JAW - BROKEN OR DISLOCATED

A broken jaw is a break in the jaw bone. A dislocated jaw means the lower part of the jaw has moved out of its normal position at one or both joints where the jaw bone connects to the skull (temporomandibular joints).

Considerations

A broken or dislocated jaw usually heals completely after treatment. However, the jaw may become dislocated again in the future.

Complications may include:

- Airway blockage
- Bleeding
- Breathing blood or food into the lungs
- Difficulty eating (temporary)
- Difficulty talking (temporary)
- Infection of the jaw or face
- Jaw joint (TMJ) pain and other problems
- Problems aligning the teeth

Causes

The most common cause of a broken or dislocated jaw is injury to the face. This may be due to:

- Assault
- Industrial accident
- Motor vehicle accident
- Recreational or sports injury

Symptoms

Symptoms of a dislocated jaw include:

- Bite that feels "off" or crooked
- Difficulty speaking
- Drooling because of inability to close the mouth
- Inability to close the mouth
- Jaw that may protrude forward
- Pain in the face or jaw, located in front of the ear on the affected side, and gets worse with movement
- Teeth that do not line up properly

Symptoms of a fractured (broken) jaw include:

- Bleeding from the mouth
- Difficulty opening the mouth widely

- Facial bruising
- Facial swelling
- Jaw stiffness
- Jaw tenderness or pain, worse with biting or chewing
- Loose or damaged teeth
- Lump or abnormal appearance of the cheek or jaw
- Numbness of the face (particularly the lower lip)
- Very limited movement of the jaw (with severe fracture)

First Aid

A broken or dislocated jaw requires immediate medical attention because of the risk of breathing problems or significant bleeding. Call your local emergency number or local hospital for further advice.

Hold the jaw gently in place with your hands while traveling to the emergency room. A bandage may also be wrapped over the top of the head and under the jaw. However, such a bandage should be easily removable in case you need to vomit.

If breathing problems or heavy bleeding occurs, or if there is severe facial swelling, a tube may be placed into your airways to help you breathe.

DISLOCATED JAW

If the jaw is dislocated, the health care provider may be able to place it back into the correct position using the thumbs. Numbing medications (anesthetics) and muscle relaxants may be needed to relax the strong jaw muscles.

The jaw may need to be stabilized. This usually involves bandaging the jaw to keep the mouth from opening widely. In some cases, surgery may be needed to do this, particularly if repeated jaw dislocations occur.

After dislocating your jaw, you should not open your mouth widely for at least 6 weeks. Support your jaw with one or both hands when yawning and sneezing.

FRACTURED JAW

Temporarily bandaging the jaw (around the top of the head) to prevent it from moving may help reduce pain. The specific treatment for a fractured jaw depends on how badly the bone is broken. If you have a minor fracture, you may only need pain medicines and to follow a soft or liquid diet for a while. Surgery is often needed for moderate to severe fractures. The jaw may be wired to the teeth of the opposite jaw to improve stability. Jaw wires are usually left in place for 6 - 8 weeks. Small rubber bands (elastics) are used to hold the teeth together. After a few weeks, some of the elastics are removed to allow motion and reduce joint stiffness.

If the jaw is wired, you can only drink liquids or eat very soft foods. Have blunt scissors readily available to cut the elastics in the event of vomiting or choking. If the wires must be cut, consult a health care provider promptly so they can be replaced.

MANDIBULAR FRACTURE

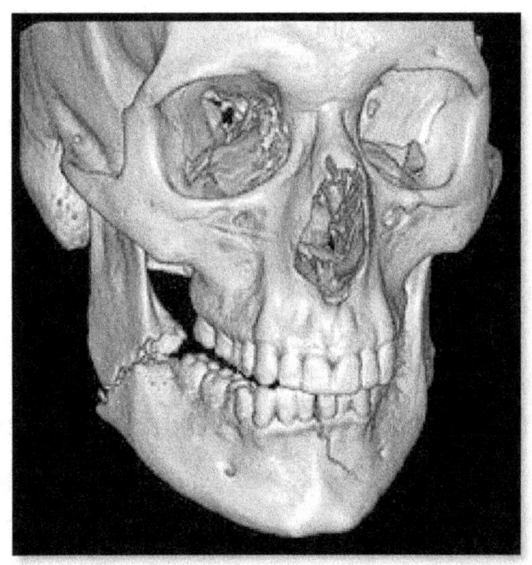

3D computed tomographic image of a bilateral mandible fracture (displaced right angle fracture involving impacted wisdom tooth and left parasymphyseal fracture).
Mandibular fracture, also known as fractures of the jaw, are breaks through the mandibular bone. They usually occur due to trauma and are often associated with other facial trauma. The types of mandibular fractures include fractures at the symphyseal area, horizontal ramus, mandibular angle and condylar neck.

Classification

There are various classification systems of mandibular fractures in use.

Location

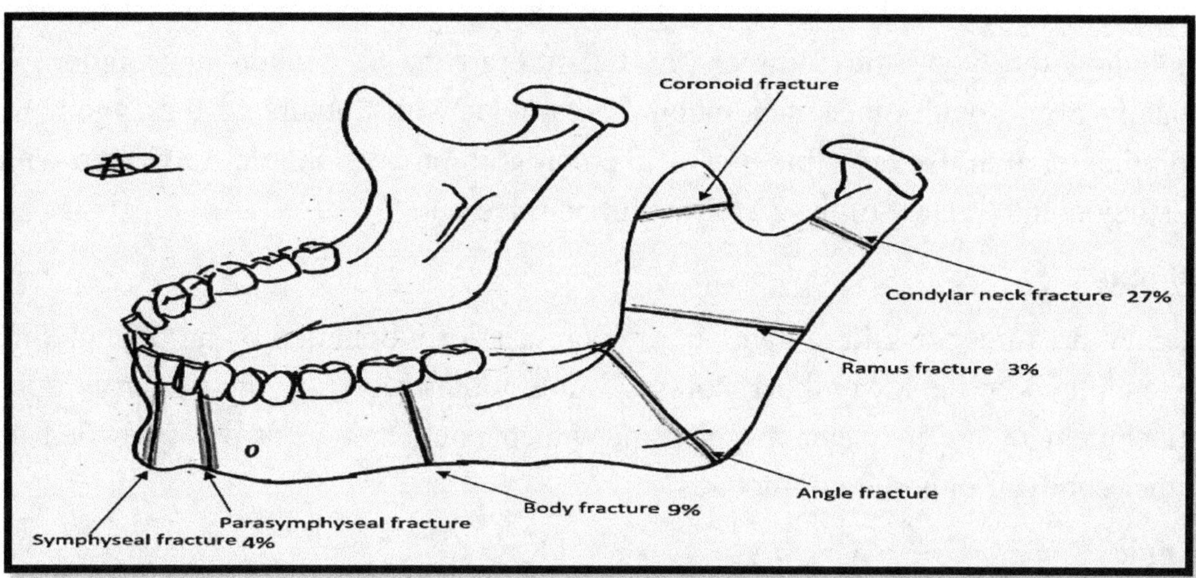

Photo of the mandible demonstrating the frequency of mandibular fractures by location.

This is the most useful classification, because both the signs and symptoms, and also the treatment are dependent upon the location of the fracture. The mandible is usually divided into the following zones for the purpose of describing the location of a fracture (see diagram): condylar, coronoid process, ramus, angle of mandible, body (molar and premolar areas), parasymphysis and symphysis.

Alveolar

This type of fracture involves the alveolus, also termed the alveolar process of the mandible.

Condylar

Condylar fractures are classified by location compared to the capsule of ligaments that hold the temporomandibular joint (intracapsular or extracapsular), dislocation (whether or not the condylar head has come out of the socket (glenoid fossa) as the muscles (lateral pterygoid) tend to pull the condyle anterior and medial) and neck of the condyle fractures. E.g. extracapsular, non-displaced, neck fracture. Paediatric condylar fractures have special protocols for management

Coronoid

Because the coronoid process of the mandible lies deep to many structures, including the zygomatic complex (ZMC), it's rare to be broken in isolation. It usually occurs with other mandibular fractures or with fracture of the zygomatic complex or arch. Isolated fractures of the coronoid process should be viewed with suspicion and fracture of the ZMC should be ruled out.

Ramus

Ramus fractures are said to involve a region inferiorly bounded by an oblique line extending from the lower third molar (wisdom tooth) region to the posteroinferior attachment of the masseter muscle, and which could not be better classified as either condylar or coronoid fractures.

Angle

The angle of the mandible refers to the angle created by the arrangement of the body of the mandible and the ramus. Angle fractures are defined as those that involve a triangular region bounded by the anterior border of masseter muscle and an oblique line extending from the lower third molar (wisdom tooth) region to the posteroinferior attachment of the masseter muscle.

Body

Fractures of the mandibular body are defined as those that involve a region bounded anteriorly by the parasymphysis (defined as a vertical line just distal to the canine tooth) and posteriorly by the anterior border of the masseter muscle.

Parasymphysis

Parasymphyseal fractures are defined as mandibular fractures that involve a region bounded bilaterally by vertical lines just distal to the canine tooth.

Symphysis

Symphyseal fractures are a linear fracture that run in the midline of the mandible.

Fracture type

Mandibular fractures are also classified according to categories that describe the condition of the bone fragments at the fracture site and also the presence of communication with the external environment.

Greenstick

Greenstick fractures are incomplete fractures of flexible bone, and for this reason typically occur only in children. This type of fracture generally has limited mobility.

Simple

A simple fracture describes a complete transection of the bone with minimal fragmentation at the fracture site.

Comminuted

The opposite of a simple fracture is a comminuted fracture, where the bone has been shattered into fragments, or there are secondary fractures along the main fracture lines. High velocity injuries (e.g. those caused by bullets, improvised explosive devices, etc...) will frequently cause comminuted fractures.

Compound

A compound fracture is one that communicates with the external environment. In the case of mandibular fractures, communication may occur through the skin of the face or with the oral cavity. Mandibular fractures that involve the tooth-bearing portion of the jaw are by definition compound fractures, because there is at least a communication via the periodontal ligament with the oral cavity and with more displaced fractures there may be frank tearing of the gingival and alveolar mucosa.

Involvement of dentition

When a fracture occurs in the tooth bearing portion of the mandible, whether or not it's dentate or edentulous will affect treatment. Wiring of the teeth helps stabilize the fracture (either during placement of osteosynthesis or as a treatment by itself), so the lack of teeth will guide treatment. When an edentulous mandible (no teeth) is less than 1 cm in height (as measured on panoramic radiograph or CT scan) addition risks apply because the blood flow from the marrow (endosseous) is minimal and the healing bone must rely on blood supply from the periosteum surrounding the bone. If a fracture occurs in a child with mixed dentition different treatment protocols are needed.

Other fractures of the body, are classified as open or closed. Because fractures that involve the teeth, by definition, communicate with the mouth this distinction is largely lost in mandible fractures. Condylar, ramus, coronoid process and ramus fractures are generally closed whereas angle, body and parasymphsis fractures are generally open.

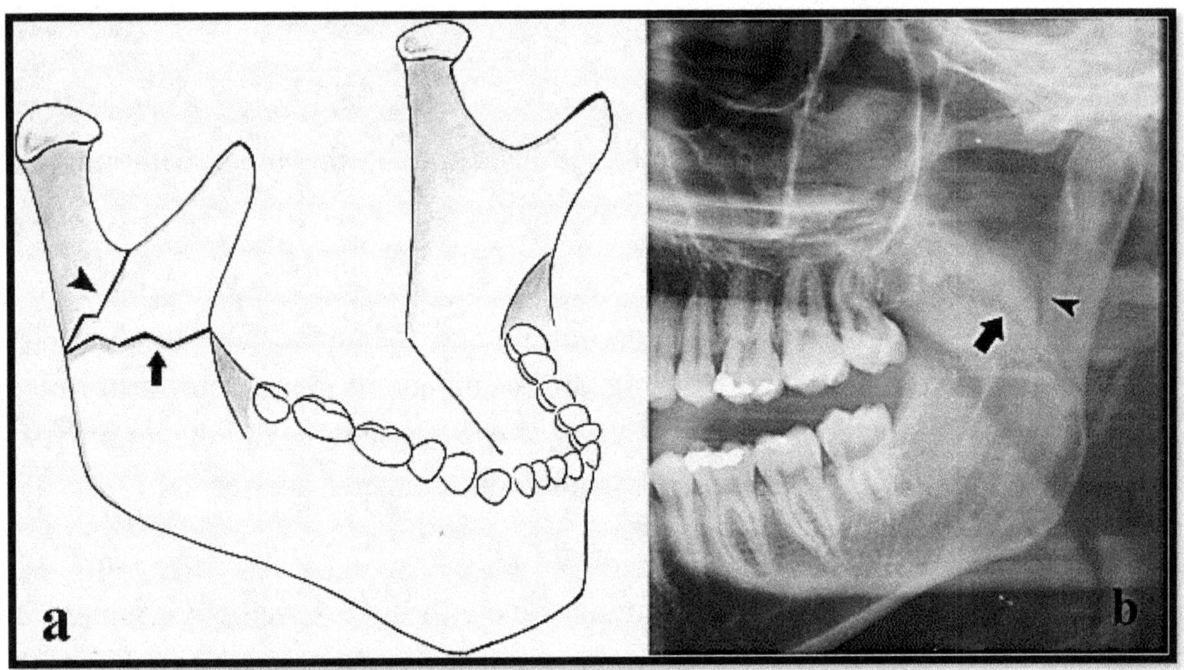

multiple mandible fractures of a patient in the right condyle (extracapsular/neck/not dislocated), right body (vertically unfavourable) and left coronoid process

Displacement

The degree to which the segments are separated. The larger the separation, the more difficult it is to bring them back together (approximate the segments)

Favorablity

For angle and posterior body fractures, when the angle of the fracture line is angled back (more posterior at the top of the jaw and more anterior at the bottom of the jaw) the muscles tend to bring the fracture segments together. This is called favorable. When the angle of the fractures is pointing to the front, it's unfavorable.

Age of the fracture

While mandible fractures have similar complication rates whether treated immediately or days later, older fractures are believed to have higher non-union and infection rates although the data on this makes it difficult to draw firm conclusions.

Signs and symptoms

General

By far, the two most **common symptoms** described are pain and the feeling that teeth no longer correctly meet (traumatic malocclusion, or disocclusion). The teeth are very sensitive to pressure (proprioception), so even a small change in the location of the teeth will generate this sensation. Patients will also been very sensitive to touching the area of the jaw that is broken, or in the case of condylar fracture the area just in front of the tragus of the ear.

Other symptoms may include loose teeth (teeth on either side of the fracture will feel loose because the fracture is mobile), numbness (because the inferior alveolar nerve runs along the jaw and can be compressed by a fracture) and trismus (difficulty opening the mouth).

Outside the mouth, signs of swelling, bruising and deformity can all be seen. Condylar fractures are deep, so it's rare to see significant swelling although, the trauma can cause fracture of the bone on the anterior aspect of the external auditory meatus so bruising or bleeding can sometimes be seen in the ear canal. Mouth opening can be diminished (less than 3 cm). There can be numbness or altered sensation (anesthesia/paraesthesia in the chin and lower lip (the distribution of the mental nerve).

Intraorally, if the fracture occurs in the tooth bearing area, a step may seen between the teeth on either side of the fracture or a space can be seen (often mistaken for a lost tooth) and bleeding from the gingiva in the area. There can be an open bite where the lower teeth, no longer meet the upper teeth. In the case of a unilateral condylar fracture the back teeth on the side of the fracture will meet and the open bite will get progressively greater towards the other side of the mouth.

Sometimes bruising will develop in the floor of the mouth (sublingual eccymosis) and the fracture can be moved by moving either side of the fracture segment up and down. For fractures that occur in the non-tooth bearing area (condyle, ramus, and sometimes the angle) an open bite is an important clinical feature since little else, other than swelling, may be apparent.

Condylar

This type of fractured mandible can involve one condyle (unilateral) or both (bilateral). Unilateral condylar fracture may cause restricted and painful jaw movement. There may be swelling over the temporomandibular joint region and bleeding from the ear because of lacerations to the external auditory meatus. The hematoma may spread downwards and backwards behind the ear, which may be confused with Battle's sign (a sign of a base of skull fracture), although this is an uncommon finding so if present, intra-cranial injury must be ruled out. If the bones fracture and overlie each other there may be shortening of the height of the ramus. This results in gagging of the teeth on the fractured side (the teeth meet too soon on the fractured side, and not on the non-fractured side, i.e. "open bite" that becomes progressively worse to the unaffected side). When the mouth is opened, there may be deviation of the mandible towards the fractured side. Bilateral condylar fractures may cause the above signs and symptoms, but on both sides. Malocclusion and restricted jaw movement are usually more severe. Displacement of the condyle through the roof of glenoid fossa and into the middle cranial fossa is rare.

Epidemiology

Mandible fracture causes vary by the time period and the region studied. In North America, blunt force trauma (a punch) is the leading cause of mandible fracture where as in India, motor vehicle collisions are now a leading cause. On battle grounds, it's more likely to be high velocity injuries (bullets and shrapnel). Prior to the routine use of seat belts, airbags and modern safety measures, motor vehicle collisions where a leading cause of facial trauma. The relationship to blunt force trauma explains why 80% of all mandible fractures occur in males. Mandibular fracture is a rare complication of third molar removal, and may occur during the procedure or afterwards. With respect to trauma patients, roughly 10% have some sort of facial fracture, the majority of which come from motor vehicle collisions. When the person is unrestrained in a car, the risk of fracture rises 50% and when an unhelmeted motorcyclist the risk rises 4-fold.

Diagnosis

Imaging

Plain film radiography

Traditionally, plain films of the mandible would be exposed but had lower sensitivity and specificity owing to overlap of structures. Views included AP (for parasymphsis), lateral oblique (body, ramus, angle, coronoid process) and Towne's (condyle) views. Condylar fractures can be especially difficult to identify, depending on the direction of condylar displacement or dislocation so multiple views of it are usually examined with two views at perpendicular angles.

Panoramic radiography

Panoramic radiographs are tomograms where the mandible is in the focal trough and show a flat image of the mandible. Because the curve of the mandible appears in a 2-dimensional image, fractures are easier to spot leading to an accuracy similar to CT except in the condyle region. In addition, broken, missing or maligned teeth can often be appreciated on a panormic image which is frequently lost in plain films. Medial/lateral displacement of the fracture segments and especially the condyle are difficult to gauge so the view is sometimes augmented with plain film radiography or computed tomography for more complex mandible fractures.

Computed tomography

Computed tomography is the most sensitive and specific of the imaging techniques. The facial bones can be visualized as slices through the skeletal in either the axial, coronal or sagittal planes. Images can be reconstructed into a 3-dimensional view, to give a better sense of the displacement of various fragments. 3D reconstruction, however, can mask smaller fractures owing to volume averaging, scatter artifact and surrounding structures simply blocking the view of underlying areas.

Research has shown that panoramic radiography is similar to computed tomography in its diagnostic accuracy for mandible fractures and both are more accurate than plain film radiograph. The indications to use CT for mandible fracture vary by region, but it does not seem to add to diagnosis or treatment planning except for comminuted or avulsive type fractures, although, there is better clinician agreement on the location and absence of fractures with CT compared to panoramic radiography.

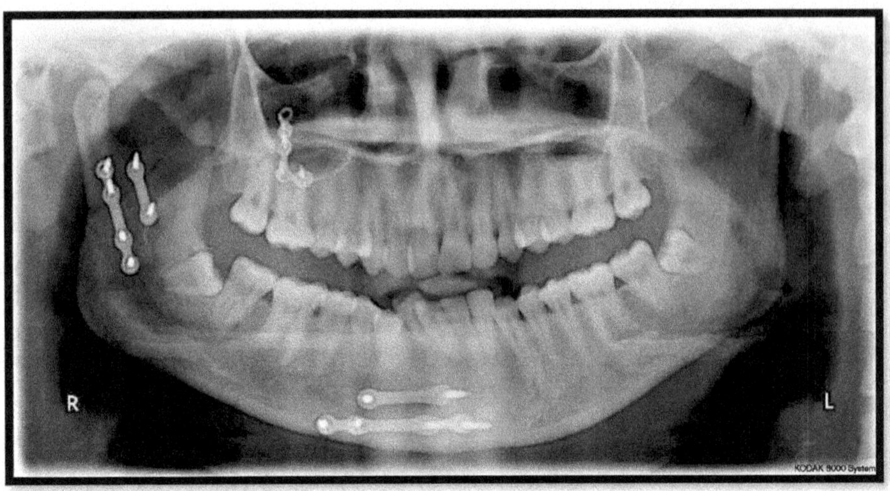

Panoramic radiograph of a simple mandible fracture of the right mandibular body, minimally displaced. Note that the teeth to the left of the fracture do not touch

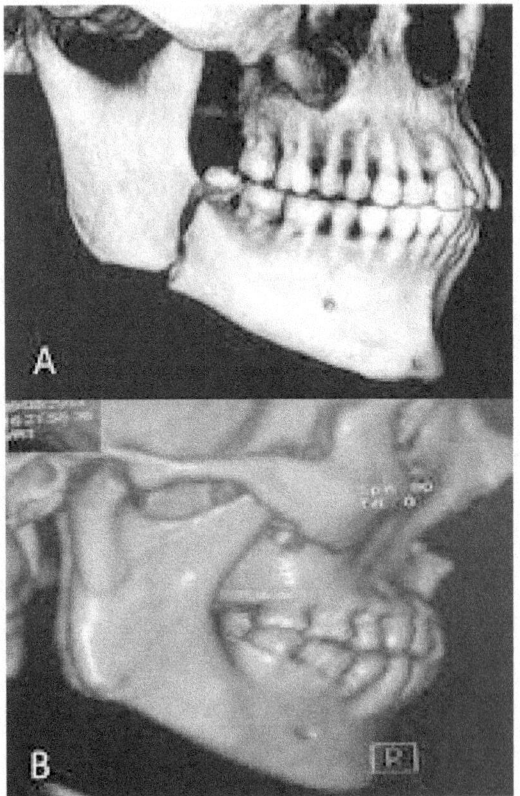

lateral oblique image demonstrating a fractured mandible

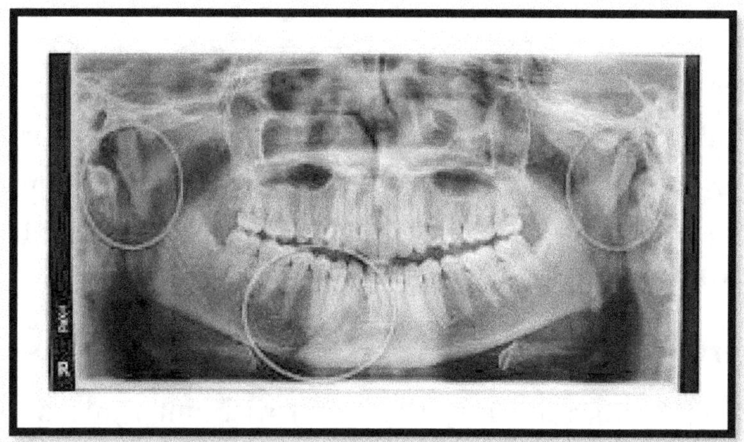

Towne's view of a bilateral condyle fracture. White arrow is a fracture on the neck of the condyle. Black arrow shows the condyle pulled to the medial. The same injury can be seen on the opposite side

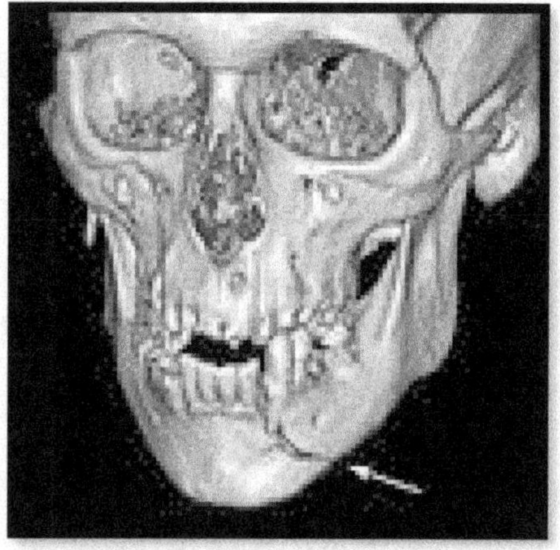

3D CT reconstruction of mandible fracture

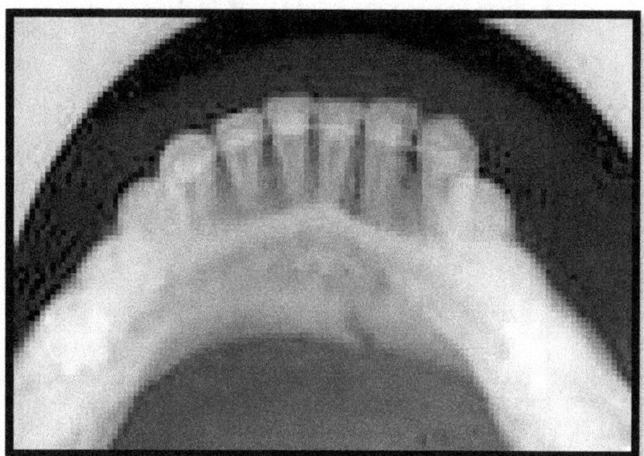

Occlusal radiograph of a mandibular parasymphasis fracture

Treatment

Like all fractures, consideration has to be given to other illnesses that might jeopardize the patient, then to reduction and fixation of the fracture itself. Except in avulsive type injuries, or those where there might be airway compromise, a several day delay in the treatment of mandible fractures seems to have little impact on the outcome or complication rates.

General Considerations

Since mandible fractures are usually the result of blunt force trauma to the head and face, other injuries need to be considered before the mandible fracture. First and foremost is compromise of the airway. While rare, bilateral mandible fractures that are unstable can cause the tongue to fall back and block the airway. Fractures such as a symphyseal or bilateral parasymphyseal may lead to mobility of the central portion of the mandible where genioglossus attaches, and allow the tongue to fall backwards and block the airway. In larger fractures, or those from high velocity injuries, soft tissue swelling can block the airway.

In addition to the potential for airway compromise, the force delivered to break the jaw can be great enough to either fracture the cervical spine or cause intra-cranial injury (head injury). It is common for both to be assessed with facial fractures.

Finally, vascular injury can result (with particular attention to the internal carotid and jugular) from high velocity injuries or severely displaced mandible fractures.

Loss of consciousness combined with aspiration of tooth fragments, blood and possibly dentures mean that the airway may be threatened.

Reduction

Reduction refers to approximating the ends of the bones edges that are broken. This is done with either an open technique, where an incision is made, the fracture is found and is physically manipulated into place, or closed technique where no incision is made.

The mouth is unique, in that the teeth are well secured to the bone ends but come through epithelium (mucosa). A leg or wrist, for instance, has no such structure to help with a closed reduction. In addition, when the fracture happens to be in a tooth bearing area of the jaws, aligning the teeth well usually results in alignment of the fracture segments.

To align the teeth, circumdental wiring is often used where wire strands (typically 24 gauge or 26 gauge) are wrapped around each tooth then attached to a stainless-steel arch bar. When the maxillary (top) and mandibular (bottom) teeth are aligned together, this brings the fracture segments into place. Higher tech solutions are also available, to help reduce the segments with arch bars using bonding technology.

Fixation

Simple fractures are usually treated with **closed reduction and indirect skeletal fixation**, more commonly referred to as **maxillo-mandibular fixation (MMF)**. The closed reduction is explained above. The indirect skeletal fixation is accomplished by placing an arch bar, secured to the teeth on the maxillary and mandibular dentition, then securing the top and bottom arch bars with wire loops.

Many alternatives exist to secure the maxillary and mandibular dentition including resin bonded arch bars, Ivy loops (small eyelets of wires), orthodontic bands and MMF bone screws where titanium screws with holes in the head of them are screwed into the basal bone of the jaws then secured with wire.

Closed reduction with direct skeletal fixation follows the same premise as MMF except that wires are passed through the skin and around the bottom jaw in the mandibule and through the piriform rim or zygomatic buttresses of the maxilla then joined together to secure the jaws. The option is sometimes used when a patient is edentulous (has no teeth) and rigid interal fixation cannot be used.

Open reduction with direct skeletal fixation allows the bones to be directly mandipulated through an incision so that the fractured ends meet, then they can be secured together either rigidly (with screws or plates and screws) or non-rigidly (with transosseous wires). There are a multitude of various plate and screw combinations including compression plates, non-compression plates, lag-screws, mini-plates and biodegradable plates.

External fixation, which can be used with either open or closed reduction uses a pin system, where long screws are passed through the skin and into either side of a fracture segment (typically 2 pins per side) then secured in place using an external fixator. This is a more common approach when the bone is heavily comminuted (shattered into small pieces, for instance in a bullet wound) and when the bone is infected (osteomyelitis).

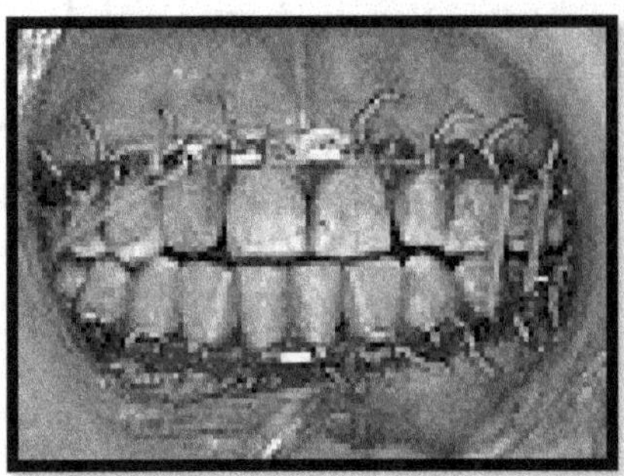

Maxillomandibular fixation with circumdental wires, archbars and elastics for a condyle fracture

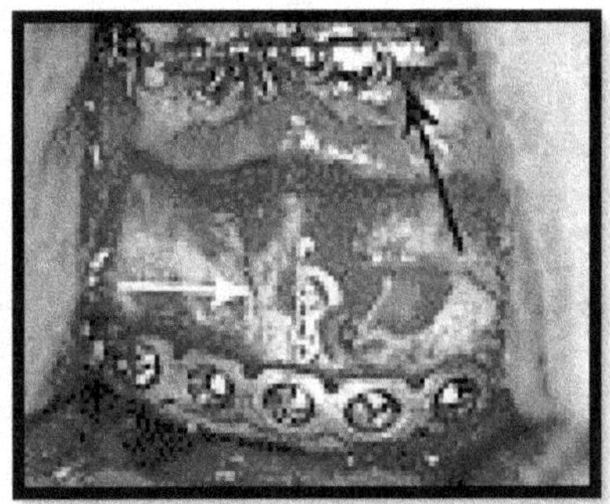

Rigid internal fixation of parasymphasis fracture of the mandible. White arrow marks fracture, black arrow marks arch bar on lower teeth

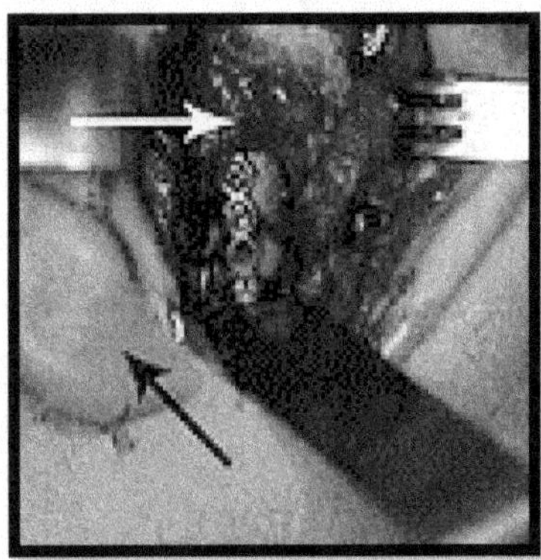

Rigid internal fixation of right condyle fracture with mini-plate on the neck of the condyle. Black arrow marks right earlobe, white arrow marks head of the condyle

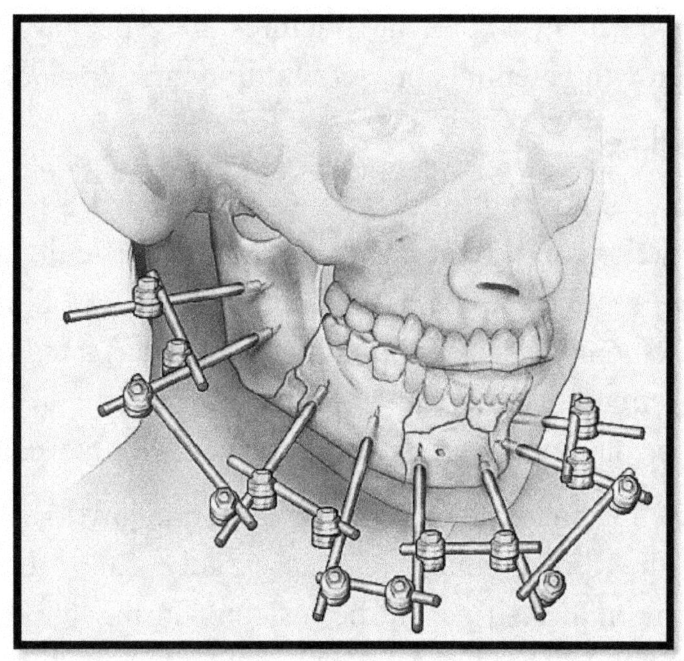

External fixation of left mandible fracture

Regardless of the method of fixation, the bone needs to remain relatively stable for a period of 3–6 weeks. On average, the bone gains 80% of its strength by 3 weeks and 90% of it by 4 weeks. There is great variation depending on the severity of injury and health of the wound and patient.

Special Considerations

Condyle

The best treatment for condylar fractures is controversial. There are two main options, namely closed reduction or open reduction and fixation. Closed reduction may involve intermaxillary fixation, where the jaws are splinted together in the correct position for a period of weeks. Open reduction involves surgical exposure of the fracture site, which can be carried out via incisions within the mouth or incisions outside the mouth over the area of the condyle. Open reduction is sometimes combined with use of an endoscope to aid visualization of fracture site. Although closed reduction carries a risk of the bone healing out of position, with consequent alteration of the bite or the creation of facial asymmetry, it does not risk temporary damage to the facial nerve or result in any facial scar that accompanies open reduction. A systematic review was unable to find sufficient evidence of the superiority of one method over another in the management of condylar fractures. Paediatric condylar fractures are especially problematic, owing to the remaining growth potential and possibility of ankylosis of the joint.

Edentulous mandible

A broken jaw that has no teeth in it faces two additional issues. First, the lack of teeth makes reduction and fixation using MMF difficult. Instead of placing circumdental wires around the teeth, existing dentures can be left in (or Gunning splints, a type of temporary denture) and the mandible fixated to the maxilla using skeletal fixation (circummandibular and circumzygomatic wires) or using MMF bone screws. More commonly, open reduction and rigid internal fixation is placed.

When the width of the mandible is less than 1 cm, the jaw loses its endosteal blood supply. Instead, the blood supply comes largely from the periosteum. Open reduction (which normally strips the periosteum during the dissection) can lead to avascular necrosis. In these cases, oral surgeons sometimes opt for external fixation, closed reduction, supraperiosteal dissection or other techniques to maintain the periosteal blood flow.

High Velocity Injuries

In high velocity injuries, the soft tissue can be severely damaged far from the bullet wound itself due to hydrostatic shock. Because of this the airway must be carefully managed and vessels well examined. Because the jaw can be highly comminuted, MMF and rigid internal fixation can be difficult. Instead, external fixation is often used.

Pathologic fracture

Fractures where large cysts or tumours are in the area (and weaken the jaw), where there is an area of osteomyelitis or where osteonecrosis exist cause special challenges to fixation and healing. Cysts and tumours can limit effective bone to bone contact and osteomyelitis or osteonecrosis compromise blood supply to the bone. In all of the situations, healing will be delayed and sometimes, resection is the only alternative to treatment.

Prognosis

The healing time for a routine mandible fracture is 4–6 weeks whether MMF or rigid internal fixation (RIF) is used. For comparable fractures, patients who received MMF will lose more weight and take longer to regain mouth opening, whereas, those who receive RIF have higher infection rates.

The most common long-term complications are loss of sensation in the mandibular nerve, malocclusion and loss of teeth in the line of fracture. The more complicated the fracture (infection, comminution, displacement) the higher the risk of fracture.

Condylar fractures have higher rates of malocclusion which in turn are dependent on the degree of displacement and/or dislocation. When the fracture is intracapsular there is a higher rate of late-term osteoarthritis and the potential for ankylosis although the latter is a rare complication as long as mobilization is early. Paediatric condylar fractures have higher rates of ankylosis and the potential for growth disturbance.

CHAPTER - 7

ASSESSMENT OF THE GASTROINTESTINAL SYSTEM

INTRODUCTION:

The gastrointestinal system (GI) consists of the GI tract and its associated organs and glands. Included in the GI tract are the mouth, oesophagus, stomach, small intestine, large intestine, rectum and anus. The associated organs are the liver, pancreas and gall bladder.

Assessing the patients with disorders of pertaining to gastrointestinal disorder is a very important task which a nurse practioner need to follow by following certain standard phenomenon. It includes collection of history and physical examination.

Evaluation of the gastrointestinal tract requires careful history and physical examination techniques. Though sophisticated laboratory tests or radiographic or endoscopic procedures may be necessary to confirm a diagnosis of intra-abdominal pathology, the initial diagnosis is usually suspected from the history and reinforced by physical examination. Most important, therapeutic decisions for intra-abdominal inflammatory processes are based mainly on findings that can be elicited only by careful physical examination. Thus, though physical examination of the abdomen is difficult, it is a skill that must be mastered for proper management of these patients.

I. Health history:

Information should be gathered from the patient about the history or the existing problems related to GI functioning is called as history collection. Collect the following information from the patient in detail,

- Demographic data

- History of travel

- Past medical and surgical history

- Current signs and symptoms

- Weight history

- Medication history (ask details if the patient is under any sort of medications)

- Past hospitalization history

- Diet history

- Food allergy

- Dietary pattern

- Activities of daily living

- Family history

- Health believes

- Sleep and rest pattern

- Role relationship pattern

- Sexuality – reproductive pattern

- Value belief pattern

- Coping stress and tolerance pattern

- Habits (ex. Alcoholism, smoking etc.,)

II. Physical examination:

The physical examination includes assessment of the GI tract from mouth to anus. The following techniques can be used to assess the GI tract,

- ❖ Inspection

- ❖ Auscultation

- ❖ Palpation

- ❖ percussion

- ❖ **Inspection:**

Looking with naked eye and assessing for the presence of any abnormality is called as inspection. Check for presence of any abnormalities including, discoloration, presence of ulcers, lesions, previous surgical scars, etc., GI assessment begins with oral cavity. The lips are examined for lesions, abnormal colour, any symmetry. The oral cavity is inspected for inflammation, tenderness, ulcers, swelling, bleeding and discoloration. Any odor of the patient is noted. The tongue should be assessed for dehydration such as dryness, cracks, or furrows. The patient's gum should be pink without swelling, redness and irregularities.

To inspect the abdomen, patients are placed in a supine position with their arms at their sides; the abdomen is visually inspected to note the condition of the skin and the contour. The contour may be rounded, flat, concave or distended depending on the patient's body type. Irregularities of the contour may be due to distention, tumours, hernia, or previous surgeries. Scars, wounds, tubes, and ostomy device type and location are noted.

Inspection findings

Inspection of the abdomen gives clues to the diagnosis of intra-abdominal pathology. Combined with the patient's history, inspection can often provide a preliminary diagnosis that can be confirmed by auscultation and palpation. Despite the current popularity of various non-invasive and invasive diagnostic tests, the experienced surgeon can usually make an accurate diagnosis of intra-abdominal pathology by history and physical examination. This is demonstrated by the patient with a several-day history of right upper quadrant and back pain with associated nausea, vomiting, fever, and a visible mass in the right upper quadrant. Such a patient almost certainly has acute cholecystitis with hydrops of the gallbladder. The remainder of the physical examination merely confirms this and detects additional disease. Though inspection alone never provides a clear diagnosis, it should not be overlooked.

Generalized distention of the abdomen is usually from obesity, bowel distention by gas or liquid, or ascites. Obesity can cause generalized distension by either fat in the abdominal wall or intra-abdominal fat in the omentum or viscera. Generalized abdominal distention can also be related to ascites, particularly when associated with an everted umbilicus. Distention of the upper half of the abdomen only may be due to pancreatic cyst or tumour or to acute gastric dilatation. Distention of the lower half of the abdomen may be due to pregnancy, ovarian tumour, uterine fibroids, or bladder distention. A scaphoid abdomen is due to malnutrition.

Skin abnormalities detected on inspection of the abdominal wall need to be correlated with the clinical history. Bruising should be correlated with a history of trauma to determine the possible organs injured. Cullen's and Grey Turner's signs (bluish discoloration of the umbilicus and flanks, respectively) are related to intra-abdominal and retroperitoneal bleeding, and it is believed the blood dissects along fascial planes to reach these areas. Thus, one would want to question the patient diligently for causes of such bleeding—severe pancreatitis, trauma, or ruptured ectopic pregnancy. Striae of the abdominal wall are a result of rupture of the reticular dermis that occurs with stretching. This is seen clinically in pregnancy, obesity, ascites, abdominal carcinomatosis, and Cushing's syndrome.

Surgical scars should be examined carefully, both as to their position and their characteristics. Often patients are unsure of what kinds of surgery they have had, but the position of the incision may give the examiner a clue. Even though a transverse right lower quadrant incision suggests appendectomy, however, it in no way proves it, and one must be circumspect in making any such assumptions. The scar tells the examiner about the surgery. All scars are initially raised and red; they gradually fade to pink and by 6 months are generally flat and skin coloured or grey. Wounds that heal cleanly by first intention are thin and regular, whereas those that are infected and heal by secondary intention are wider and irregular. Keloids are wide, irregular scars with abundant hypertrophic tissue outside the field of normal scarring. Keloid formation tends to recur in certain individuals and is particularly common in blacks.

Enlarged veins are seen in three clinical situations: emaciation, portal hypertension, and inferior vena cava obstruction. In emaciation there is loss of subcutaneous fat so that the normally invisible veins become prominent. These veins become more prominent in the presence of portal hypertension. In portal hypertension the umbilical vein becomes an outflow tract of the portal system and forms collaterals with the veins of the abdominal wall. This is responsible for the caput medusa that is diagnostic of portal hypertension. The direction of blood flow in these veins in portal hypertension is normal (i.e., upward in those above the umbilicus and downward in those below) as the blood is flowing from the high-pressure portal system to the low-pressure systemic system. Finally, the veins of the abdominal wall may be dilated due to obstruction of the inferior vena cava. This occurs because the abdominal wall becomes a collateral, or bypass, around the obstruction of the cava. In this situation the direction of blood flow will be reversed below the umbilicus as the blood flows from the femoral vein to the superior vena cava. Obstruction of the inferior vena cava can occur as a result of a hepatic malignancy, as an extension of hepatic vein obstruction (Budd–Chiari syndrome), as a result of thrombophlebitis, or as a result of trauma or surgical intervention.

Masses noted on inspection of the abdomen may be related to organs in that area. Thus, a mass in the right upper quadrant may represent hepatomegaly from hepatitis or hepatic tumour, a distended gallbladder from cholecystitis or pancreatic cancer, or a carcinoma in the head of the pancreas. An epigastric mass is likely to be from acute gastric distention. pancreatic pseudocyst, pancreatic cancer, or aneurysm of the abdominal aorta (which will be pulsatile). Masses in the left subcostal region are generally due to splenomegaly, although carcinoma of the spenic flexure of the colon is also a possibility.

Masses in the lumbar region are generally of renal origin. Renal cysts, polycystic kidneys, and renal malignancies may all be visible in asthenic patients.

Masses in the lower quadrants may result from inflammatory or neoplastic disorders of the intestine. In the right lower quadrant appendiceal abscess and caecal carcinoma are most likely, while in the left lower quadrant diverticular abscess or carcinoma of the sigmoid colon is most likely.

Hypogastric masses are the result of pelvic pathology. Acute urinary retention is the most common cause of such a mass in males. In females, uterine or ovarian neoplasms may cause visible midline abdominal masses.

Visible intestinal peristalsis is usually the result of intestinal obstruction. This can be seen in the stomach of the newborn with hypertrophic pyloric stenosis and in the small intestine of patients with small bowel obstruction from various aetiologies.

❖ **Auscultation**

Hearing the sounds of the bowel with the help of an stethoscope is called as auscultation. Before auscultating the bowel, divide the whole abdomen into nine quadrants,

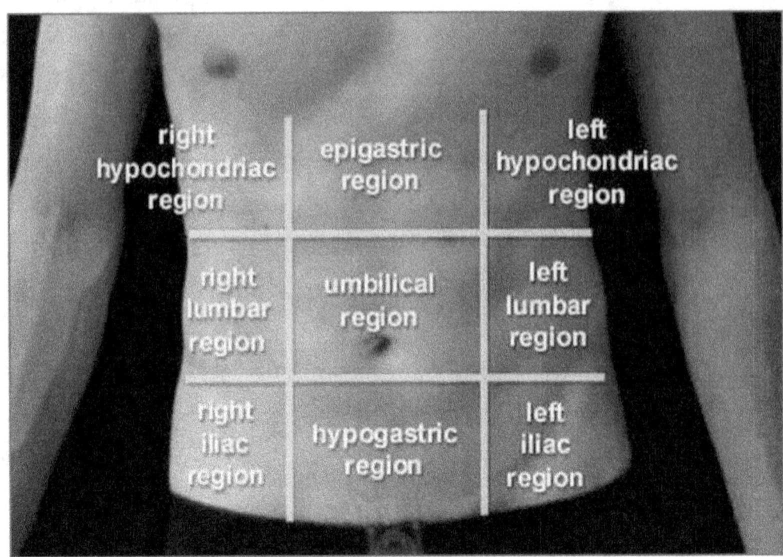

Nine quadrants

The patient is positioned comfortably in the supine position. The stethoscope is used to listen over several areas of the abdomen for several minutes for the presence of bowel sounds. The diaphragm of the stethoscope should be applied to the abdominal wall with firm but gentle pressure. It is often helpful to warm the diaphragm in the examiner's hands before application, particularly in ticklish patients. When bowel sounds are not present, one should listen for a full 3 minutes before determining that bowel sounds are, in fact, absent.

In abdominal examination auscultation is performed before palpation, as palpation may alter the bowel sounds. Starting in the right upper quadrant, the examiner listens over the liver for rubs or bruits and over the free abdominal wall for bowel sounds. One moves next to the left upper quadrant, again listening for bowel sounds and then over the spleen to detect rubs or bruits.

One should next auscultate in the periumbilical regions for aortic or renal bruits and for bowel sounds and then in the left and right lower quadrants for bowel sounds or iliac bruits. If, during the course of auscultation, no bowel sounds are detected, one should auscultate in the periumbilical region for 3 full minutes before determining that bowel sounds are absent. Important points to note on bowel sounds are the pitch, intensity, and duration of the sounds. Any bruits noted should be carefully localized to the loudest point as this relates to the origin of the bruit.

Rubs are infrequently found on abdominal examination but can occur over the liver, spleen, or an abdominal mass.

Auscultation findings

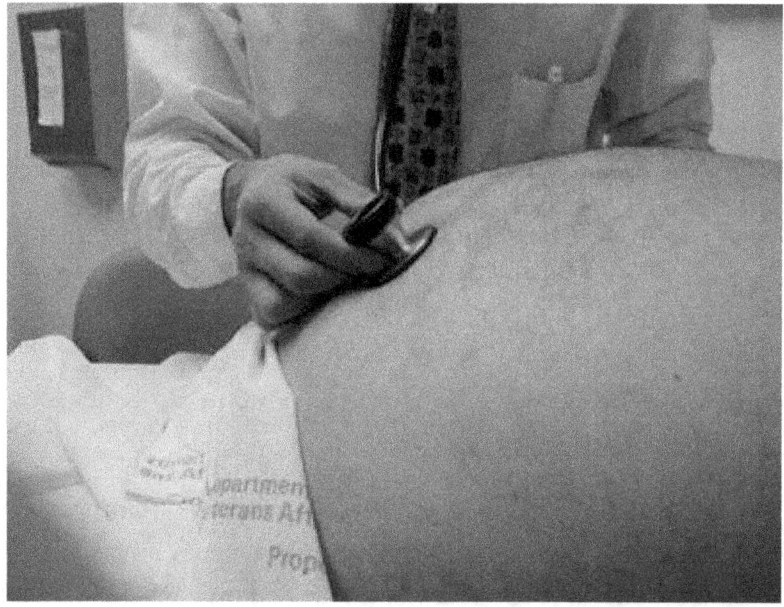

Bowel sounds are of significance to the clinician as a marker of intra-abdominal pathology. The absence of bowel sounds may be one of the few indicators of intra-abdominal infection in patients with multiple problems and, particularly, altered mental status. In patients with generalized abdominal distention following laparotomy, bowel sounds may be the key diagnostic finding to differentiate ileus from early postoperative small bowel obstruction. Though radiographic examination of the abdomen may suggest bowel obstruction, the characteristic high-pitched bowel sounds are diagnostic for the experienced clinician.

Similarly, vascular bruits are helpful to the clinician as an indicator of underlying pathology. Thus they should be carefully searched for in patients with hypertension (renal artery stenosis), chronic abdominal pain (mesenteric arterial insufficiency), or claudication (occlusive disease of the aorta or iliac arteries). As continuous bruits are caused by arteriovenous fistulas, they should be searched for carefully in patients with penetrating abdominal trauma.

Abdominal rubs are rare, but may be found over the liver or spleen. A rub implies that the surface of the organ is irregular and usually is due to involvement by tumour, abscess, or infarction. More rarely, an inflammatory intra-abdominal mass may have an associated rub caused by irritation of the adjacent abdominal wall.

❖ Palpation and Percussion

The patient is positioned supine with head and knees supported, as for Inspection and Auscultation. Take the history and perform inspection and auscultation before palpation, as this tends to put the patient at ease and increases cooperation. In addition, palpation may stimulate bowel activity and thus falsely increase bowel sounds if performed before auscultation. Ask patients with abdominal pain to point to the area of greatest pain. Then reassure them that you will try to minimize their discomfort and examine that point last.

In palpating the abdomen, one should first gently examine the abdominal wall with the fingertips. This will demonstrate the crunching feeling of crepitus of the abdominal wall, a sign of gas or fluid within the subcutaneous tissues. In addition, it will demonstrate any irregularities of the abdominal wall (such as lipomas or hernias) and give some idea as to areas of tenderness.

Deep palpation of the abdomen is performed by placing the flat of the hand on the abdominal wall and applying firm, steady pressure. It may be helpful to use two-handed palpation particularly in evaluating a mass. Here the upper hand is used to exert pressure, while the lower hand is used to feel. One should start deep palpation in the quadrant directly opposite any area of pain and carefully examine each quadrant. At each costal margin it is helpful to have the patient inspire deeply to aid in palpation of the liver, gallbladder, and spleen.

In the flanks it is often helpful to elevate the flank to be examined slightly and place one hand on the lower ribs of that flank to "push" the retroperitoneal contents up to the examining hand. In this way, small renal masses that would otherwise be missed may be appreciated.

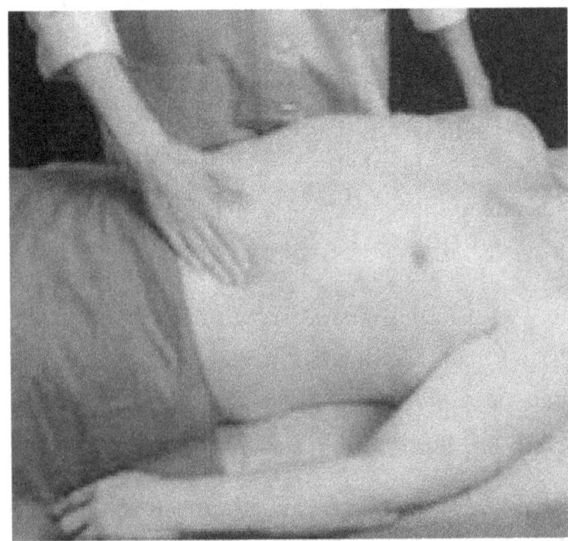

One handed palpation

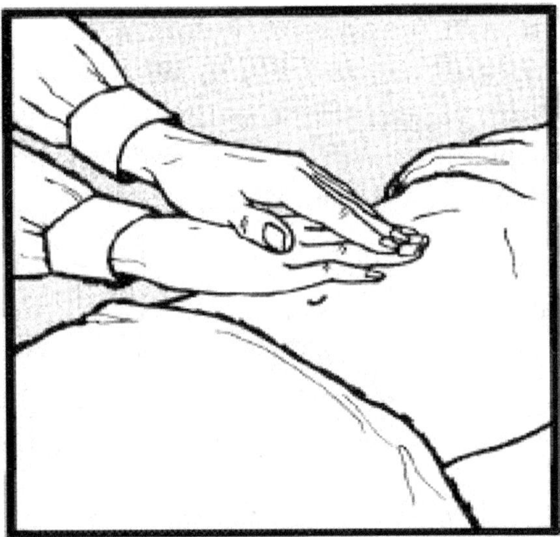

Two-handed deep palpation

Abdominal tenderness is the objective expression of pain from palpation. When elicited, it should be described as to its location (quadrant), depth of palpation required to elicit it (superficial or deep), and the patient's response (mild or severe). Spasm or rigidity is the involuntary tightening of the abdominal musculature that occurs in response to underlying inflammation. Guarding, in contrast, is a voluntary contraction of the abdominal wall musculature to avoid pain. Thus, guarding tends to be generalized over the entire abdomen, whereas rigidity involves only the inflamed area. Guarding can often be overcome by having the patient purposely relax the muscles; rigidity cannot be. Rigidity is thus a clear-cut sign of peritoneal inflammation.

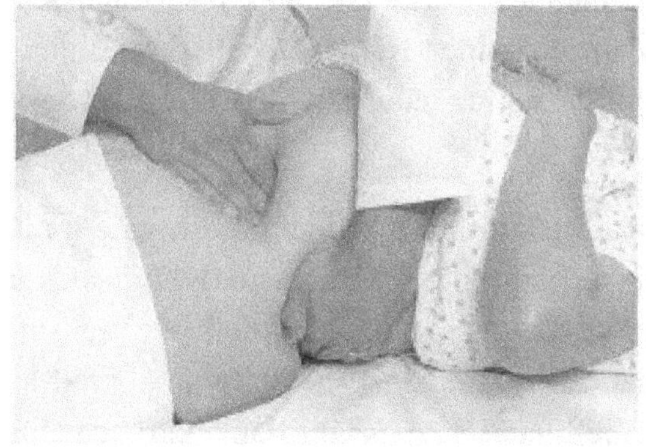

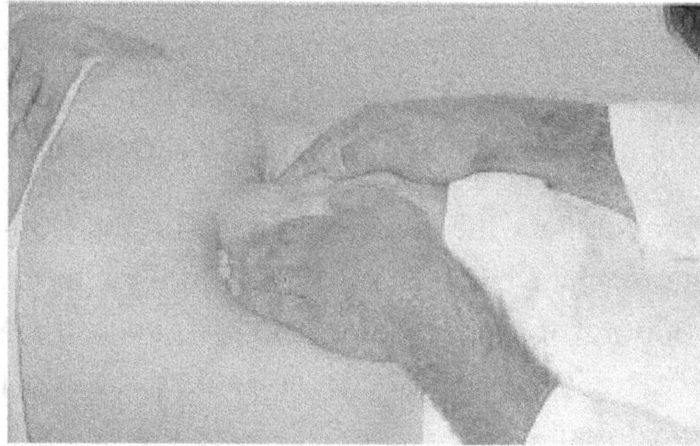

<u>Alternative hand technique</u>   **<u>Deep palpation technique</u>**

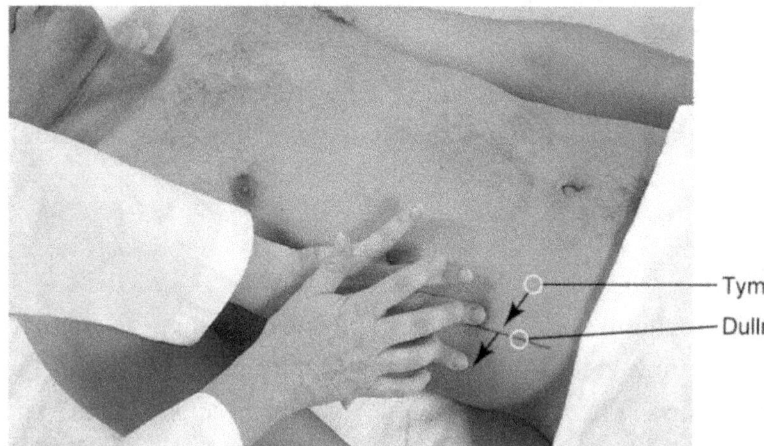

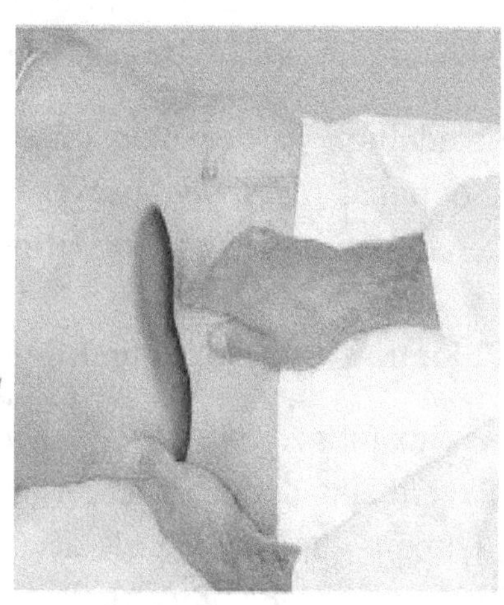

<u>Percussion</u>   **<u>Palpating appendix</u>**

Rebound tenderness is the elicitation of tenderness by rapidly removing the examining hand. Again, this is a difficult sign for the beginning examiner to master. The most common error is to remove the hand very quickly with an exaggerated motion and thus startle the patient. All that needs to be done is smoothly but quickly to lift the palpating hand off the abdomen and observe for pain, facial grimace, or spasm of the abdominal wall. Both tenderness and rebound tenderness may be elicited by palpation in a different quadrant. Thus, palpation of the left lower quadrant may produce tenderness and rebound tenderness in the right lower quadrant in appendicitis (Rovsing's sign). This is called referred tenderness and referred rebound.

When abdominal masses are palpated, the first consideration is whether the mass is intra-abdominal or within the abdominal wall. This can be determined by having the patient raise his or her head or feet from the examining table. This will tense the abdominal muscles, thus shielding an intra-abdominal mass while making an abdominal wall mass more prominent. If the mass is intra-abdominal, important points are its size, location, tenderness, and mobility.

Palpation and percussion are used to evaluate ascites. A rounded, symmetrical contour of the abdomen with bulging flanks is often the first clue. Palpation of the abdomen in the patient with ascites will often demonstrate a doughy, almost fluctuant sensation. In advanced cases the abdominal wall will be tense due to distention from the contained fluid. Gas-filled intestines will float to the top of the fluid-filled abdomen. Thus, in the supine patient with ascites there should be periumbilical tympany with dullness in the flanks.

One should mark the level of dullness on the skin and then turn the patient on one side for a full minute. A change in the level of dullness is termed shifting dullness and usually indicates more than 500 ml of ascetic fluid. Another physical sign of ascites is demonstration of a transmitted fluid wave. The patient or an assistant presses a hand firmly against the abdominal wall in the umbilical region. The examiner places the flat of the left hand on the right flank and then taps the left flank with his right hand. In the presence of ascites, a sharp tap will generate a pressure wave that will be transmitted to the left hand. Unfortunately, fat will also transmit a fluid wave, and there are frequent false-positives with this test.

In addition to detection of ascites, percussion can be used to help define the nature of an abdominal mass. Tympany of an abdominal mass implies that it is gas filled (i.e., intestine). Percussion is also used to define liver size.

Palpation and Percussion findings

As mentioned previously, abdominal tenderness is a difficult physical finding to master. Nevertheless, it is a finding that must be mastered because it is often the only clear finding in peritonitis and may well determine therapy. The classic example of this is appendicitis. The history and laboratory findings may suggest appendicitis in a patient with abdominal pain, but the presence or absence of tenderness makes or breaks the diagnosis. As there are no laboratory studies that can either exclude or ensure the diagnosis of appendicitis, the clinician must make therapeutic decisions based on the physical finding of tenderness.

As tenderness is caused by inflammation of the parietal peritoneum, the aetiology of tenderness can be related to the underlying organs. Thus, right upper quadrant tenderness may be caused by cholecystitis, ulcer disease, pancreatitis, or hepatitis. Epigastric tenderness is usually due to pancreatitis or peptic ulcer disease. Right lower quadrant tenderness may be related to appendicitis, caecal diverticulitis, or perforated carcinoma, whereas left lower quadrant tenderness is usually due to sigmoid diverticulitis. Flank tenderness is usually related to renal pathology, either pyelonephritis or perinephric abscess.

When tenderness is generalized, one must consider causes for generalized peritonitis. Acute perforated ulcer is a frequent cause and presents with characteristic "board like" rigidity of the abdominal wall. Other common causes include perforated diverticulitis, perforated appendicitis, and pancreatitis. Nevertheless, any process that produces generalized peritoneal irritation (chemical or infectious) will produce the same physical findings.

Abdominal masses are related to the underlying organs. Right upper quadrant masses include hepatomegaly, hydrops of the gallbladder, and carcinoma of the head of the pancreas. Epigastric masses are pancreatic (pseudocyst or carcinoma), gastric malignancies, and colon malignancies. Masses in the left upper quadrant are usually due to either splenomegaly or carcinoma of the stomach or colon. In the flanks, masses usually arise from the kidney (cyst or tumour), although occasionally from other retroperitoneal structures (lymphoma, sarcoma).

Masses in the lower quadrants usually arise from the bowel. On the right side, common masses include appendiceal abscess and caecal carcinoma; on the left, diverticular abscess and sigmoid carcinoma. Central abdominal masses are often aortic aneurysms, and the pulsatile nature of the mass is diagnostic. Thus, in evaluating an abdominal mass, one must consider its location, mobility, and the presence or absence of tenderness in order to define its aetiology.

The clinical significance of ascites is based largely on its aetiology. This can often be determined by the history and physical examination, but paracentesis is diagnostic. Samples of peritoneal fluid should be sent to the laboratory for protein concentration, specific gravity, cell counts, and culture. Exudative ascites occurs in bacterial peritonitis, carcinomatosis, and pancreatic ascites and is associated with a protein concentration of over 3 gm/dl and a specific gravity above 1.016. Transudative ascites occurs in cirrhosis, Budd–Chiari syndrome, constrictive pericarditis, congestive heart failure, and hypoalbuminemic disorders such as the nephrotic syndrome. In these incidences the protein concentration is less than 3 gm/dl and the specific gravity less than 1.016.

Clinical significance of physical examination

- Normal peristalsis of the intestine produces bowel sounds as gas and fluid are passed through the intestinal lumen. Normally, the bowel sounds are intermittent, low-pitched, chuckling sounds. Bowel sounds may be decreased or increased in disease states.

- Ileus is a failure of peristalsis and is the normal physiologic response of the intestine to laparotomy or peritoneal inflammation. In addition, ileus is seen in a number of disease states that do not affect the peritoneum directly, including pneumonia, congestive heart failure, and uremia. Bowel sounds will be markedly diminished or absent in ileus as the intestine distends with gas in its paralyzed state.

- Early mechanical bowel obstruction produces hyperactive peristaltic waves proximal to the mechanical obstruction. These waves are increased in frequency and force and produce a concomitant increase in bowel sounds with characteristic "rushes." As the bowel gradually dilates with gas and fluid, the bowel sounds become high pitched and tinkling, and there may be periods of hypoactive bowel sounds that alternate with hyperperistaltic rushes. These rushes correlate with the increased peristaltic activity. Finally, in late intestinal obstruction there may be loss of all bowel sounds due to loss of peristaltic activity from vascular compromise.

- Vascular bruits are the audible manifestation of turbulent blood flow. They are found normally in thin patients, but in heavier individuals will be muffled because of the surrounding fat. Loud systolic bruits are due to atherosclerotic plaques within arteries, producing turbulent flow. These plaques are common in the aorta and iliac arteries and less common in the renal arteries. In addition, turbulent flow within an abdominal aortic aneurysm may create a bruit. Bruits that are present in both systole and diastole are strongly suggestive of an arteriovenous communication.

- Rubs are uncommon on abdominal auscultation but, when found, are the result of inflamed peritoneal surfaces grating on each other during respiration. This can be the result of a neoplastic or infectious process that destroys the normally smooth peritoneal surfaces.

- Crepitus is produced by gas (air) and/or fluid within tissues. In the abdominal wall, it either is due to traumatic introduction of air or is secondary to infection (gas gangrene). Subcutaneous emphysema can occur from rupture of a pulmonary bleb or penetrating chest injury with dissection of air into the subcutaneous spaces. In addition, penetrating abdominal trauma may introduce enough air into the abdominal wall to produce crepitus. Gas gangrene can occur as a complication of intra-abdominal surgery and produce crepitus of the abdominal wall. The gas is produced by anaerobic bacteria (usually clostridia species) and is a very specific clinical sign when found in the patient with wound infection.

- Abdominal tenderness occurs as a result of irritation of the parietal peritoneum. While inflammation or irritation of the visceral peritoneum will cause abdominal discomfort, anorexia, and poorly localized pain, it will not cause tenderness and rigidity of the abdominal wall. Irritation or inflammation of the parietal peritoneum will stimulate the pain fibres of the parietal peritoneum and abdominal wall, creating the symptoms of localized pain and the signs of tenderness, rigidity, and rebound tenderness. Thus, if there is diffuse irritation of the peritoneum, as in diffuse peritonitis, there will be diffuse tenderness and rigidity.

- Abdominal masses arise from the surrounding structures, thus the importance of topographic relationships. The presence or absence of tenderness of a mass gives important information as to its etiology. An appendiceal abscess will be tender as it inflames the parietal peritoneum, whereas carcinoma of the cecum will be nontender because there is no inflammation involved. Tympany over a mass implies it is gas filled. In the abdomen, this usually signifies the mass is dilated bowel, as only rarely will there be enough gas in any other mass to produce tympany.

- Ascites is the presence of intra-abdominal fluid and occurs because of overproduction of intra-abdominal fluid or lack of absorption. It is most commonly seen in cirrhosis in which there is an increase in portal pressure and hypoalbuminemia. The increased portal pressure hydrostatically increases transudation of fluid through capillaries, whereas the hypoalbuminemia hydrostatically favours ascites formation. Thus, there is accumulation of fluid in the peritoneal space, which signifies severe liver disease.

Rectal and anus examination

The perianal and anal areas should be inspected for colour, texture, lumps, rashes, scars, erythema, fissures, and external haemorrhoids. Any lumps at the unusual areas should be palpated. Ask the patient to turn to the left lateral decubitus position with the right hip and knee fully flexed and the left hip and knee slightly flexed. The gluteal region should be at the edge of the examining table. The anal area is then carefully examined for any skin lesions, scars, fistula tracts, or external haemorrhoids. The gloved right index finger is then well lubricated and inserted anally. Resistance at the anal ring is usually due to spasm caused by nervousness and may be overcome by asking the patient to strain as the finger is inserted. The anal wall is carefully palpated, taking note of any hypertrophic, inflamed crypts, strictures, and for sphincter tone. The fingertip then palpates the rectum to check for any rectal mass and for the condition of the prostate.

Inguinal Region

Examination of the inguinal region is best performed by having the patient stand erect facing the examiner who is seated on a stool. The examiner should inspect the inguinal region for evidence of abnormal protrusions or masses along the course of the spermatic cord into the scrotum. If a suspicious mass is detected on inspection, the patient should be asked to cough to see if any additional impulse occurs. He should be asked to attempt to reduce the mass himself if that is possible.

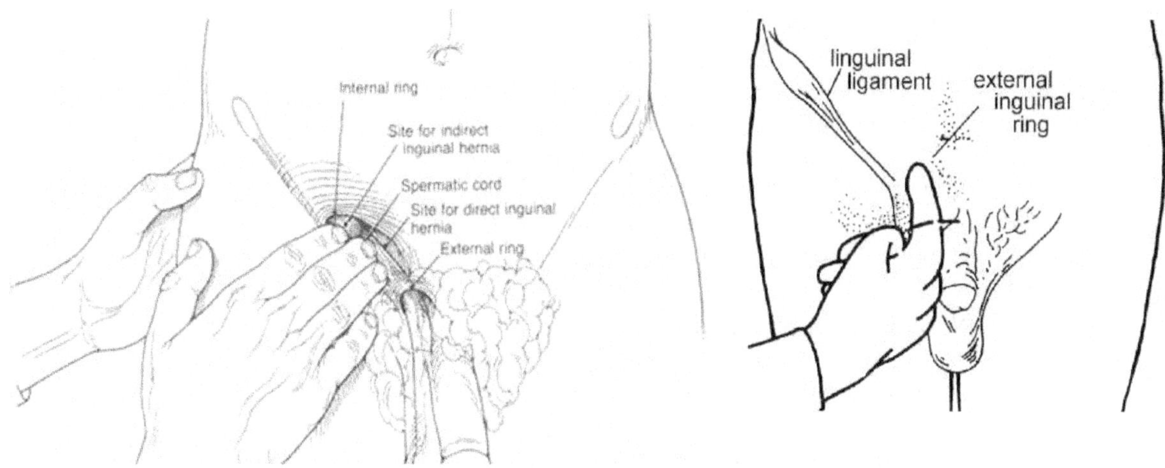

<u>**Palpating the inguinal region**</u>

If no mass is evident, the examiner should palpate the inguinal regions. This is best done by inserting the index finger along the spermatic cord inverting the scrotal skin to the pubic tubercle and then sweeping laterally to identify the external ring. The subject is then instructed to cough, and if an indirect inguinal hernia is present, the examiner should detect an impulse as the sac proceeds along the inguinal canal to exit at the external ring. If a general bulge is detected in the medial inguinal region, differentiation between direct and indirect inguinal hernia occasionally can be made on physical examination by pressing directly over the internal ring and thereby arresting descent of the indirect hernia. If the subject then coughs again and the same protrusion occurs with the internal ring occluded, one can assume that the hernia is a direct hernia through the lower abdominal wall.

Summary of normal physical assessment of GI system

Region	Findings
Mouth	<ul><li>Moist and pink lips</li><li>Pink and moist buccal mucosa and Gingiva without plaques or lesions</li><li>Teeth in good repair</li><li>Protrusion of tongue in midline without deviation and fasciculation</li><li>Pink uvula in midline, soft palate, tonsils and posterior pharynx</li><li>Swallows smoothly without coughing or gagging.</li></ul>
Abdomen	<ul><li>Flat without mass or scar</li><li>No abdominal tenderness</li><li>No bruises</li><li>Bowel sounds in all quadrants</li><li>Non palpable liver and spleen</li><li>Liver 10 cm in midclavicular line</li><li>Generalized tympany</li></ul>

Anus	• Absence of lesions, fissures and haemorrhoids
	• Good sphincter tone
	• Rectal wall smooth / soft
	• No masses
	• Stool soft / brown / heme negative

COMMON ASSESSMENT OF ABNORMALITIES OF GASTROINTESTINAL SYSTEM

Findings	Description	Possible aetiology and significance
Mouth : • Ulcer, plaque on lips / mouth • Cheilosis • Cheilitis • Geographic tongue • Smooth tongue • Leukoplakia • Pyorrhea • Herpes simplex • Candidiasis • Glossitis • Gingivitis	• Sore or lesion • Softening, fissuring and cracking of lips at the angles of the mouth. • Inflammation of lips with fissuring, scaling and crusting. • Scattered red, smoth areas on dorsum of tongue. • Red, slick appearance • Thickened white patches • Recessed gums, purulent pockets • Benign vesicular lesions	• Carcinoma, viral infections • Riboflavin deficiency • Often unknown • Cobalamin deficiency • Premalignant lesion • Peritonitis • Herpsevirus • Candida albicans • Irritation, infury, vit, B deficiency • Ill-fitting dentures, food impaction

	• White curd like lesion around ertythematous mucosa • Reddened, ulcerated, swollen tongue. • Edematous, painful and bleeding gingivae.	
Esophagus and stomach: • Dysphagia • Hematemesis • Pyrosis • Dyspepsia • Odynophagia • Eructation • Nausea and vomiting	• Difficulty in swallowing • Vomiting of blood • Heart burn • Burning or indigestion • Painful swallowing • Belching • Feeling of impending vomiting	• Oesophageal problem, ca of oesophagus • Oesophageal varices, bleeding peptic ulcer • Hiatal hernia, esophagitis • Peptic ulcer and gall bladder disease • Ca of oesophagus and esophagitis • Gallbladder disease • GI infection, stress, fear, pathologic condition.
Abdomen: • Distention • Ascites • Bruit • Hyperresonance • Borborygmi • Absent bowel sound	• Gas accumulation and enlarged abdomen • Accumulated fluid within the abdominal cavity • Humming or swishing sound heard from abdomen • Loud, tinkling rushes • Waves of loud, gurgling sound	• Obstruction, paralytic ileus • Peritoneal inflammation, heart failure, metastatic cancer, cirrhosis • Partial arterial obstruction, aneurysm • Intestinal obstruction • Hyperactive bowel as a result of eating

• Absence of liver dullness • Masses • Rebound tenderness • Nodular liver • Hepatomegaly • Splenomegaly • Hernia	• No auscultation of bowel sounds • Tympany on percussion • Lump on palpation • Sudden pain when fingers withdrawn quickly • Enlarged hard liver with irregular edges • Enlarged liver &edges >1-2 cm below costal margin • Enlargement of spleen • Bulge or nodule in the abdomen	• Peritonitis, paralytic ileus, obstruction • Air from viscus (e.g., perforated ulcer) • Tumours, cyst • Peritoneal inflammation, appendicitis • Cirrhosis, carcinoma • Hepatitis, venous congestion • Chronic leukaemia, portal hypertension, infection • Defect in the muscle.
Rectum and Anus: • Haemorrhoids • Mass • Pilonidal cyst • Fissure • Melena • Tenesmus • Steatorrhea	• Thrombosed veins in the rectum and anus • Firm, nodular edge • Sinus tract, cyst in midline just above coccyx • Ulceration in anal canal • Black, tarry stool containing digested blood • Painful and ineffective straining of stool • Fatty, frothy- smelling stool	• Portal hypertension, chronic constipation, infection • Tumour, carcinoma • Probably congenital • Straining, irritation • Cancer, bleeding ulcer and varices • Ulcerative colitis, food poisoning • Chronic pancreatitis, biliary obstruction, malabsorption problem.

GASTROINTESTINAL ASSESSMENT FORMAT

I. PATIENT'S PROFILE

Name of the patient   :

Age   :

Sex   :

Ward   :

Unit   :

MRD number   :

Marital Status   :

Educational Qualification   :

Religion   :

Occupation   :

Family income   :

Address   :

Source/ informant   :

Date of admission   :

Date of surgery   :

Number of post operative day :

Medical diagnosis   :

Reason for Hospitalization   :

II. HISTORY OF PRESENT ILLNESS

Mode of onset, cause of disease and details of treatment, detailed symptoms with special emphasis on chronological order according to the sequence of events (for example fever for the past one week) self-medicated treatment (duration, site, severity radiation, associated features ex fever nausea).

III. PAST HEALTH HISTORY

From birth to till now – history of illness, surgery, injury and methods of treatment (drugs and blood transfusion), allergies to drugs, status of immunization, H/o exposure of STDs previous similar episodes.

IV. FAMILY HISTORY

- Type of family

- Determine the risk factors among the family members

- History of cardiac disease, hypertension, diabetic mellites, jaundice, mental illness, congenital abnormalities, communicable disease among the family members

- Draw the Genogram.

V. SOCIO ECONOMIC HISTORY

Type of housing   :

Own/rented   :

Water facility   :

Drainage facility   :

Cross ventilation   :

Disposal of refuse   :

Lighting facility   :

Pet animals   :

Garden   :

VI. PERSONAL HISTORY

- Place of birth

- Personal experience at different ages

- Relationship with neighbourhood and family

- Values, beliefs, practices on religious factors

- Language spoken and understood

- Food types and values (in detail)

- Patterns of rest and sleep

- Social and recreational preferences

- Smoking/drug abuse/alcohol

- Activities of daily living.

VII. MENSTRUAL HISTORY (For female patients)

- Age at Menarche

- Menstrual cycle

> *Number of days/month
> *Regular/ irregular
> *Painful bleeding or not

VIII. MARITAL HISTORY

- Age at marriage

- Consanguineous marriage with degree

IX. OBSTETRICAL HISTORY (For female patients):

S. No	Order of birth	Term/preterm	Mode of delivery	Place of birth	Birth attendant	sex of the baby	Weight of the baby	Health status

PHYSICAL ASSESSMENT:

General appearance: body built (well-built, moderately built, thin built),

Well-groomed/dull/ depressed/ anxious/oriented to

Time place person

Hair and scalp   :   Distribution of hair/colour of hair/ texture/

infestations(pediculi/dandruff)

Eyes   :   Vision(normal/refractory errors/discharges/colour

                             Of the cornea/colour of inferior palpabrae of the

                             Conjunctiva/ abnormalities(ptosis)

Ears   :   Hearing(normal/ hard of hearing)/discharges

                             Symmetry/asymmetric/low set ears/cerumen

                             Accumulation

Nose   :   Septal deviation(Present/absent discharges) bleeding

Mouth and throat :   Lips- colour/ inflammation/dry/ normal

                             Stomatitis/odour/breath odour/lesions

                             Tongue- clean/coated/colour glossy/glossitis

                             Dry/moist/bleeding gums/ sore mouth/ abscess/

                             Teeth –alignment(normal/ mal aligned)/dental

                             Carries/ uses of dentures/ partial plates/ last dental

                             examination/ results

Throat   :   Inflammation/tonsils(normal/ enlarged)

                             Halitosis./ difficulty in swallowing/ presence or

                             absence of tonsils/ abscess/hoarseness of voice

Neck   :   Normal/ short/ torticollis/stiffness/ thyroid gland

                             Enlargement/ lymph node enlargement

Chest   :   Symmetry/bilateral air entry/ movement on respiration

Abdomen: Contour(scaphoid/sausage/flat/pendulous/distended)

                             Abdominal aorta pulsation distension (Don't touch

                             during inspection phase it may induce peristalsis)

Genitalia   :   Swelling/un descended testis/ulcers/discharges/

                             Position of urinary meatus

Upper and lower extremities: Range of motion/ swelling/muscle wasting/

Congenital abnormalities/ colour of nail beds/ clubbing shortening of limbs

Back and spine   :   Normal curvature/ kyphosis/ scoliosis/lordosis/

pressure ulcers.

SYSTEMIC REVIEW

Central nervous system : GCS/ memory/ mood and affect

Respiratory system :

Observation - Symmetry, chest movements on respiration, rate, cough, Dyspnoea.

Auscultation - Breath sounds -vesicular breath sounds/ rales/rhonchi/adventitious

Percussion   - Resonance(normal /dull/ hyper)

Cardiovascular System :

Inspection   - Pulse(rate, volume, abnormalities)

Auscultation -   Apical heart rate, heart sounds(normal/murmur

Percussion   - Resonance (normal/dull)

Gastrointestinal System:

Inspection   - Contour of abdomen, symmetry, abdominal aorta pulsation

Abdominal distension,

Auscultation - Bowel sounds in all four quadrants(hyperactive/

High-pitched/gurgling/ clicking/ Frequency (5 to 15 times /mt is

normal) Hypo active/ Hyper active (should check for 5 minutes in

each quadrant) Vascular sounds (best heard with bell of diaphragm)

listening bruits (Aortic pulsation may be heard over the left upper

quadrant in the presence of hypertension, aortic insufficiency or

aortic aneurysm) Diminished, normal.

Percussion : Tympani- It should predominant as air rises to surface of the

abdominal cavity.

Hyper resonance - Will be heard in the presence of gaseous distension.

Dullness - Percussed over a distended bladder, adipose tissue, fluid

or a moss in the abdomen.

Palpation: (Make the patient to flex the knees to relax the abdominal

muscles. Ask the patient to point to any pain or tender area. Save those

areas to palpate last so the patient doesn't guard throats the exam.

Lightly palpate the abdomen by quadrants Note muscle guarding

rigidity, tenderness or masses).

Organomegaly: presence of lump(shape size, hardness, irregular margin,

nodularity, consistency)

Bowel movements - present/absent

Stools: Diarrhoea/constipation/colour/odour/frequency

Rectum :   Examine external rectal area for presence of external

haemorrhoids, masses, or evidence of inflammation

Musculoskeletal system:

Bulk/tone/power/peripheral pulses

Range of motion (normal/ restricted/impossible)

Congenital abnormalities shortening of limbs/Paresis/paralysis.

Endocrine system : Hot& cold intolerance/ glutition test(positive / negative)

Diabetic mellitus (known/untested)

Lymphatic system   : Generalized lymphadenopathy/local lymphadenitis

Genito-urinary system : Ulcers / swelling/ infectious/discharges/ position

Urinary meatus (in males) undescended testis

Bladder movements (frequency/ incontinency/ urgency)

dysuria/dribbling/hesitancy) total urine output Per day

Integumentary system : Turgor/ complexion/ temperature/ inflammation

Pigmentation/paraesthesia

VITAL SIGNS:

Temperature   :

Pulse   :

Respiration   :

Blood pressure   :

Pain   :

O^2 saturation   :

Gastrointestinal system and its structural and functional abnormality may affect the entire function of an individual. So utmost care must be taken to diagnose the disease conditions which affect the GI tract. To achieve this knowledge of physical assessment of the GI tract is very essential for the medical and paramedical professionals.

REFERENCES

- Lakhwindar Kaur, 2012, A Text Book of Nursing Foundation, Bangaluru, Pee Vee Publications.

- Kozier and Erb's, 2009, Fundamentals of Nursing, Philadelphia, Pearson Publications.

- Lewis, 2012, Text Book of Medical Surgical Nursing, Mosby Publications.

- Ohashi A, Tamada K, Wada S, et al. Risk factors for recurrent bile duct stones after endoscopic papillary balloon dilation: long-term follow-up study. Dig Endosc.

- Gurusamy K, Sahay SJ, Burroughs AK, Davidson BR. Systematic review and meta-analysis of intraoperative versus preoperative endoscopic sphincterotomy in patients with gallbladder and suspected common bile duct stones. Br J Surg.